A Guy's Guide
to Throat Cancer

Do's and Don'ts for Recovery

Edmund A Rossman III

ISBN 978-1-0980-1533-6 (paperback)
ISBN 978-1-0980-1534-3 (digital)

Christian Faith Publishing, Inc.
832 Park Avenue
Meadville, PA 16335
www.christianfaithpublishing.com

Printed in the United States of America

Backstory

This story begins with telling you about my sister Elizabeth, aka Betty or B because our very young nieces had problems pronouncing her name, henceforth, calling her Aunt B, and me, Uncle E! You know how adorable little kids' mistakes can "B," and how they make their way into a family's history forever.

In the fall of 2017, Betty came down with an inoperable brain tumor. It was not discovered at once, but the nature of her symptoms required her to have 24-7 care. She was born with just one kidney and had complicated medical issues due to the tumor including a physical imbalance that made her dizzy and unable to go upstairs. Finally after stays in various hospitals and nursing homes, when we pressed to have a scan for a concussion injury, it was discovered that she had a brain tumor. She had chemotherapy treatments over the course of three months, going back and forth for overnight stays at the hospital and nursing home between August and December.

Betty had just started her twenty-fourth year as a teacher for the Parma School district. She was also busy as a volunteer at Our Lady of Angels Parish and had friends and family throughout the country concerned about her. She was never a big social media person, but she did use it for a short while in the first month. However, the tumor started acting on her cognitive and physical functions, and did not stop despite the chemo treatments. Betty had dozens of friends and colleagues who were concerned with her and always anxious for any updates. She eventually was settled into a nice nursing home in Parma in her school district, making access easier for her school buddies but was down at the main campus of University Hospitals in

Cleveland several times. All in all, she was in three different nursing home and six different hospital rooms in the course of four months.

We as a family did our best relaying what was going on, which hospital she was at, where to send cards, and where and when she could have visitors. It was challenging to say the least, but we managed.

About half way through this, in early November, I was diagnosed with throat cancer. To be specific, oropharyngeal cancer. I could never pronounce it right, so I just call it throat cancer. The tumor in my neck was removed on November 30, and the biopsy a few days later confirmed it was stage 4B oropharyngeal cancer. I'd need a combination of chemo and radiation treatments. Stage 4C cancer would've been terminal, so I dodged the bullet there.

Betty ended up passing away on December 30, 2017, less than a year after we had suddenly lost our mother Eleanor on January 5, 2017. Our impromptu network was efficient at getting the sad news out, and over one hundred fifty friends and family were able to come to Betty's services, despite the cold Cleveland winter.

Due to the nature of our circumstances, my doctors, Dr. Shah and Mendpara, said I could postpone treatment a little while but had to get started by mid-January. I put in for an FMLA leave for twelve weeks starting then. When discussing with my co-workers the communication challenge we had with Betty, my supervisor, Cindy, asked if I'd ever heard of CaringBridge. CaringBridge is a social media closed platform, meaning I as a patient would control who could have access. People use it to send out an update once instead of five or six times like we did with Betty, hoping we didn't forget anyone. I checked it out and thought *Man, this would've been great to have with B!*

So I registered for it, invited my Facebook friends and others to subscribe and started sending out posts. In essence, journaling my battle with cancer. Many of my network had just gone through the trauma of losing my sister, just on the heels of losing my mother who had, at age eighty-six, been the last of her generation and the matriarch of our family. It was especially hard on my father, who I am named for, after losing his wife of sixty years to lose his eldest daughter and now faced with possibly of losing his eldest son. I didn't want to compound anyone's grief or worry, so I made most of the posts pretty upbeat. CaringBridge also allows for replies to my posts like Facebook, and once I figured out how that worked I really enjoyed their comments. When my battle was over and I'd won (for now), many people told me they were glad I was healthy, but they'd miss my posts! So for all my friends and family who supported me, I say thanks, and this book is my way of paying back the love you showed.

The format is simple. First my raw CaringBridge entries, then the 'Extended version' (which for songs like Gimme Shelter if you google them, the extended versions are way cooler), my commentaries on the situation I would tell people about in person or on the phone and more descriptive of the various videos I used since the reader probably has not seen the same ones. My dad is not into computers that much so I would go into the CaringBridge descriptions with him, making him laugh and bolstering his spirits as much as he would do the same for me.

The Bible quotes are from a monthly religious magazine called *The Word*, which has the readings from every day's Roman Catholic mass. As I was a "shut-in" for almost three months straight, outside of going to treatments, I got into the routine of reading that day's Old Testament, Psalms, New Testament, and gospel readings. As you will see many times they applied to what was happening to me. Those coincidences were more than mere coincidences to me and showed me God was looking out for me, not letting my spirit grow weak, as I'm sure Mom and Betty were too.

I'm in remission now as I begin this in November of 2018. My only regret is I didn't post more, but I didn't realize God would have me use my passion for writing to get this story out despite having chemo-brain and some memory lapse. This story is not just for my friends and family but to all the guys and their caregivers, who are facing the same ordeal. Don't let pity or pride wall you off from your friends and family. Take it one day at a time, always looking for the good, the funny, the encouraging sounds and signs that point toward the joy of living.

"When cancer kicks you in the —, have it kick you forward!"

My Story

January 20, 2018

Welcome to my CaringBridge website. I'm using it to keep family and friends updated in one place. I appreciate your support and words of hope and encouragement. My chemo and radiation treatments for throat cancer begin on Monday, January 22. Chemo drug is Cisplatin and takes about six hours to be applied, followed that day by a ten-minute blast of radiation. Chemo will also be done on February 12 and March 9. Radiation treatments will be everyday Mondays to Fridays until March 9. After that, the radiation resonates against the cancer without the beam for three to four weeks. I had a food tube placed in me on January 16, kind of reminds me of being a Borg from *Star Trek*. Also I had a medical port, which was placed inside my chest on January 17 so they don't keep pricking my veins for the chemo, blood draws, etc. The University Hospital team is very impressive. I also have a nutritionist and speech therapist that'll help me keep swallowing correctly. I got plaster casts of my teeth today, which are used to create "tooth trays." I'll use for fluoride treatments twice a day and plan to use them as paperweights! Stephen King would be proud, ha ha.

Extended version:

When I heard I might never taste anything again, naturally I was a bit PO'd. What would life be like without being able to taste a great beer, burger…, fill in the blank for your own appetite. So just to be sure, I scheduled a second opinion with the best doctor I could find in the city treating this disease. Thanks to Google and the fact that I live in Cleveland—home of many fine hospital systems and all very competitive—I zeroed in on one and arranged for a review of my condition. My hospital sent all my diagnostic material, even slides of my biopsy, to this other doctor. He concurred on what my condition was and the treatment regimen. He did not agree on putting in a port or food tube unless I really required it.

He and I had a difference on balancing the "threshold of pain" and the risk of infection from the extra equipment. The port saved my arm from becoming a pincushion. As you'll see ahead, chemotherapy doesn't require only one injection of liquid plutonium (which basically is what it is) but several injections of various things. As if I didn't have enough problems, I didn't want to add "Nurses trying painfully hard to find a vein" to the pile of trouble I was facing.

He also would not recommend putting in a food tube unless it "really got bad" swallowing. It's all well and good trying to tough things out. Yes, it'd be really macho being independent of the tube and trying to swallow enough nutrition to stay healthy. But I'm a terrible cook, live independently, and couldn't see NOT taking the prophylactic precaution of having a source of nutrition inserted in my stomach prior to wasting away from hunger and having to go through that medical procedure halfway into my other treatments. I can't imagine having that procedure when my immune system was already down or getting up and down from the radiation table for a couple of weeks while the soreness went away, not to mention having my body to learn to sleep another way so I wouldn't roll on this new thing in my chest. It was definitely worth doing in advance while I was rested and relatively healthy.

One of my favorite books on working out is *Burn the Fat, Feed the Muscle* by Tom Venuto. He talks about progressive increments to build muscle. In the first week of training, doing easy sets of weights to get your body accustomed to the movements, then progressively increasing the weight load. These pretreatment precautionary measures were like that for me. They were some serious medical procedures—getting me acclimated to the hospital atmosphere, prepping my body for a more rigorous experience. The port and my food tube were weird, true that, but were also my aces in the hole down the line.

I mentioned Stephen King because as most of my family and friends know, I'm a huge fan. One of my plans for being off work was to catch up on all the movies and old books of his I hadn't done in a while. Little did I know how drained I was going to be. If I'd have a buck for every time I fell asleep while watching TV or reading, I'd be able to buy the *Browns*!

Journal Entries

1. Tested and Ready

January 20, 2018

Yes, last week was all pretreatment tests and fittings, and next week the treatment begins.

Oh and yes, this site is ready too! Thank you to my beta-testers, Tom, Ann, and Kathy, who checked it out on various devices!

They said in one of the prep classes to keep a diary, it helps to prevent chemo-brain, so I'll be posting various things (won't get too graphic) that I go through or have found inspiring…tunes, quotes, etc.

Today's the feast day of Saint Fabian, a pope and martyr from around 250 A.D. A scripture reading from Wisdom 10:12 was used in the entrance antiphon that seemed appropriate to the moment *"The Lord granted him a stern struggle that he might know that godliness is more powerful than anything else."*

Comments:

Annie A.

Hey Ed, talked to Stark girls tonight and the Nuns at SJA Convent (St. Joseph's Academy-my sisters' high school) already have you on their prayer list. Lotsa Prayer Warriors out there for you!!! xoxo

Mary O'D.

Hello Eddie—We are praying for you and know you are STRONGER than your diagnosis and you are going full force to be cured of it. We would love to help you in any way that you need and are here for you. Go kick some ass!!!

John—your favorite cousin

Hey cousin, Thinking of you. Can they pour beer in the feeding tube?

Extended version:

I had two surgical treatments and one radiation "fitting" the week before treatments started.

On Tuesday, January16, I had my "food tube" inserted. It was an all-day procedure that I had to fast for. They're very thorough about asking questions about who you are and when you were born. Every doctor, nurse, and anesthesiologist did this, which was a little annoying, but better than making them mistake me for a colonoscopy patient. Leaving my brother, Tom, in the waiting area after getting prepped with a surgical gown, they prepped me for a few hours with drugs designed to get my body ready for the anesthesia and surgery, then they wheeled me through the corridors to the surgery room, which was fun after being in a curtained-off bed area for two hours. The crew had just come back from lunch, and I was glad they'd be more focused on me rather than their *Subways* (the hospital main food franchise, one of my favorites too) They BS'd with me for a few minutes, explained I'd be asleep shortly and before I could scoff at that, I was gently being woke up in the curtained bed area again, except this time with a large bandage just south of my solar plexus. Tom came in, and we hung out for a long couple of hours. When the time came for me to start moving, a special nurse came in to explain a girdle like wrap they wanted me to wear to help stabilize and protect the tube. This tube comes out about four to five inches from the body, and if left loose, it would hang over my stomach just below the belly button. I never left it loose because it would pull at the top and feel like it could slip out! I got rid of the girdle after the first few days and became an expert at taping it close to the body. Should've shaved first though; that would've kept me from some needless hair tugging!

Surprisingly the next day they scheduled for the port placement. This was in another part of the same hospital but did not require fasting or getting knocked out. It took about four hours, comprised of an hour of waiting, getting prepped, the procedure, then post-op waiting. Tom took me there too. I had the funniest trio of nurses. They could've been right out of a Seinfeld skit, making cracks about each other, their friends, and families almost nonstop! They also were playing a pop radio station and when they weren't chatting, one would be singing. I only needed a local anesthetic, but the procedure required some ultrasound and other *Star Trek* type of targeting diagnostics. The port is about an inch wide or so, and I carry a card in my wallet that explains technically what it is in case I'm in an accident and emergency crews need to know what type of device it is, how it can be used, etc. The procedure is basically cutting me open, securing the port to my upper chest area, and feeding a tube into one of my major blood vessels to distribute whatever drugs or hydration I'm being given. It's an easy target but requires some training and the right equipment to use. It is better than constantly pricking my arms, looking for veins. It is like using a soft-nosed dart and dartboard instead of the more traditional hard-steel darts and corkboard.

In the '90s I started one of the first websites in Cleveland as business manager of alternative radio station WENZ-FM *The End*. After Clear Channel bought us and I was laid off, I started teaching for Kent State's Journalism School and working at Lakewood Library's Technology Center. I worked on a lot of internet projects, so naturally knew the value of testing platforms before a big launch. I'm really glad my team gave CaringBridge a thumbs up!

And speaking of teams, I'm glad my sister Ann and girlfriend Kathy accompanied me to the chemo class! We went about two weeks before chemo started, and frankly I forgot a lot of the details.

It is not a bachelor-friendly lesson plan. There was a lot of talk about germs, using hand sanitizer, a soft toothbrush, baby shampoo, not exactly manly stuff. They also discussed moisturizers a lot. Almost everyone's head in the class (fifteen women, two guys including me) bounced like bobble heads when the instructress discussed products like Lubriderm, Aveeno, Vaseline Intensive Care, not to mention fun brands like imodium for diarrhea, milk of magnesia, and dulcolax for constipation. I was blissfully ignorant going into this talk, but as you'll see later on, I had major painful complications with some of these conditions. It's called learning the hard way. Avoid that if possible! During post-treatment, my workmates and friends did say I looked a lot better than they expected. Aquaphor was recommended for my neck region, where I had daily radiation treatments. It did start turning red like a severe sunburn, but thanks to my nurses nudging me and Kathy and Ann slathering the stuff on me, the damage never really got too painful and went away quickly. Thank God for women!

> "*Whatever you do in life, surround yourself with smart people who'll argue with you*" (John Wooden).

The prep class in hindsight was pretty useful. They got me to stock up on things like Gatorade and yogurt, hydration-oriented food with vitamins like citruses. I took the advice of a lot of nutritional suggestions as if preparing for a marathon or an iron-man race, which in a way I was.

Chemo-brain was a term I'd heard and always just a joke I used when taking cold medicine. It's not a joke anymore. It's a form of what I call dementia—affecting memory, attention, discipline, verbal discourse, and the ability to learn. Thank goodness, the hospital had this great "chemo class" that taught me physical things like what metrics they use to watch your health and response to treatment. Things like white blood cell counts and platelets as well as the aforementioned hygiene and nutritional advice. And thank goodness, friends and family could join me in it because as I was being treated, much of the advice faded like background noise to me.

The Bible quote I used is also letting guys (and anyone) know that there will be a tough struggle ahead, and all the scientific prep in the world won't matter without faith and acting in a godly way—that is in observance of His laws and reverence for the role models that God and Jesus present to us. Jesus didn't indulge in pity on Calvary. He did have family and friends there to support him even if it was just bearing witness.

2. EZ Does It

January 22, 2018

It was a long day, but I am glad to get the first chemo and radiation treatment out of the way. I was in an easy chair throughout the day, watching the news, reading, snacking, slipping blue Powerade, not a bad life, haha.

I was apprehensive though. In the morning I heard this rocking tune I had in my head all day, a motivating call to arms. It was *Walk on Water!* by Thirty Seconds to Mars.
Celebrated by having a Heath shake from Steak and Shake!

Comments:

Audrey J.

Smart man. Never underestimate the healing powers of a Steak & Shake milkshake!

Kimberly P.

I had no idea that Ed was dealing with this until recently. That's why I hadn't seen him at the library for some time. He's a sweet person who has a warm personality toward all of us at the library. I wish Ed a speedy recovery and stay strong, because all of us are standing in his corner. ED ROSSMAN STRONG!!!

Extended version:

"Do you believe that you can walk on water? Do you believe that you can win this fight tonight?"
Thirty Seconds To Mars, Walk On Water

That was the chorus from this song. All the shots in the video were filmed in one day on July 4, 2017, but I didn't know that as I was being driven to my first chemo treatment. I just loved the timing of hearing it and the attitude it expressed.

The day in chemo went from 8:45a.m. to 3:15 p.m. Kathy drove me and assembled a picnic-type bag with yogurt, Gatorade, nutri-bars, and some cut-up fruit. The staff also served lunch. I think I tried a turkey sandwich. Thanks for not remembering, chemo-brain!

Of course everyone's treatment will be different, but here's the timeline of how mine went. The biggest shocker to me was the variety of preparatory fluid injections there were and how only a little time the actual Cisplatin treatment was. We're dealing with liquid pluto-nium here; I guess that's for the best. It obviously had its impact! As you'll see from the variety of hoses they needed for the entire chemo treatment, I'm REALLY glad I had the medical port. About ten were needed that they otherwise would've been sticking into my arm veins for…

8:45 a.m.—*A saline solution containing potassium and magnesium for two hours*
10:45 a.m.—*A saline solution with lasix, a diuretic and two tabs of compazine, plus another bag of Aloxi for an hour*
11:45 a.m.—*Decadron, a steroid to fight anti-nausea, dexamethasone, about fifteen minutes between the two bags (sounds like a George Burns joke…I was in chemo, stuck between two bags)*
12:00 p.m.—*Emend, also to fight nausea, and mannitol, a kidney pro-tector, also for about fifteen minutes*
12:15 p.m.—*Cisplatin, 225mg worth. The nurses were dressed in bio-logical warfare outfits to administer this. They had all been wear-ing mouth masks anyway because it was January, the height of flu*

season, and obviously both the patients and pro's needed all the protection they could get. But the seriousness of seeing them don the Andromeda Strain-type outfits told me we were getting down to the serious nitty-gritty for an hour.

1:15 p.m.—A posttreatment hydration time, straight saline for two hours
3:15 p.m.—I was released!

The hospital made us as comfortable as possible. The chemo class had actually ended with a tour of the Infusion Center where the treatment would be. We were in a two-person cubicle with a really comfortable lounge chair, TV and remote for each side, curtain if we wanted privacy, and for the Cisplatin application, and chairs or benches for visitors. They even had an "oven" where they kept heated blankets! I didn't indulge at first but would as the day went on…and on…and on…

I also learned how to disconnect the stand-up intravenous unit from the monitoring electronics power source (they also had backup batteries) and walk to the local men's room. More on that walk later! I fought hard to contain the dragon and not make that walk, but then I realized in the last two hours that I needed the Cisplatin out of me, that's why they give all the diuretics and saline hydration. So I gave in and sure enough, I started making the walk every twenty minutes or so.

Fresh air after being released tapped down the urge for a bit. My weight was about two hundred thirty, I could stand to lose a little water weight. However, afterward I did want to celebrate a little so we went to a drive-through restaurant that offered discount craft shakes until 4:00 p.m. I rarely was able to take advantage of it because of work. It tasted great and little did I know how soon it would be when I would not be able to enjoy it again!

I expected the chemo treatment to be more of a battle that initial time than it was. Overall it was a pleasant day, thanks to the steroids! Even that night I was feeling good. However, I followed the doctor's orders and did not go out to mix it up with friends at a bar to brag about my first treatment. Posing like Rocky when he was getting slugged by Clubber Lang and kept saying, "Aint so bad, Ain't so bad," after each punch. I stayed in and waited to see what they predicted would be an inevitable crash once the steroids wore off.

DO YOU BELIEVE THAT YOU CAN WALK ON WATER? DO YOU BELIEVE THAT YOU CAN WIN THIS FIGHT TONIGHT?

In Matthew 14:22–34, Jesus was seen walking on the water in a storm, toward the disciples in a boat. Peter (to confirm that Jesus was not a ghost) asked that he would come out to him if it is truly him. Jesus said yes, and miraculously Peter got out of the boat and walked on water himself. However, he's distracted by the storm, lost focus on Jesus, and started slipping under the waves, crying for help. Jesus saved him and mildly chastised him, asking, "Why did you lose faith?"

Belief in the buoyancy of Christ can give anyone the power to persevere and create miracles themselves. Walking over the waves of chemicals being placed in the body, supported by the faith in God that there will be a good outcome of all this, can turn the tide of fear into one of optimism and as Nicholas Murray Butler said (in a quote a friend gave me in a plaque), "Optimism is the foundation of courage." The power to overcome adversity (as my dad liked to say in closing conversations with his fellow police officers) comes to those who "keep the faith." Jesus told Peter and the disciples in the boat, keep the faith, and you too can do miracles. You too can walk on water and win this fight!

3. Rockin' Radiation

January 23, 2018

For my second day of radiation, I heard Journey already playing in the room…I don't know if they had it on for my sake or theirs, but I asked them to leave it on. Funny, I don't like the band that much, but I know all the words to their hits! And I knew I'd have that tight mask on for only about two songs, which did go by quick. I told them about my background in radio briefly and said, "We'll have to rock out again tomorrow!" Two other patients were in the waiting room. They were very chop-chop there, very efficient.

> Don't stop believin', hold on to that feelin'
> Journey, Don't Stop Believing

Comments:

Jim R.

Hi Eddie—Glad a Journey tune helped smooth the way. Saw Star Wars tonight in Brooklyn on the big screen. Thought of you! May the force be with you. Cousin Jim

Stephanie T.

Hi Ed, I miss you at Woods tonight. Our Simone brought delicious peanut cookies and potatoes chips, I will eat one for you. Stay joyful through your journey. You're in my thoughts and prayers.☺♥♥

Extended version:

Going under the radiation gun typically causes apprehension in everyone, I'm sure. The radiology team I had were excellent. One had even remembered me from my church; we had a mutual friend whom I used to teach with and who worked the church fish fries as well as a reader at the Sunday masses! Hate to say it, there was a time when I attended more fish fries in a year than masses. Anyway, it was nice of her to recognize me, put a little normalcy into a surreal situation.

The hospital must've taken a survey and found that patients loved heated blankets! Here was another department who had an oven and was glad to cover me up with one. For the neck radiation blast, I did have to take my upper body clothing off each time so these blankets were actually pretty practical because the room was kept a little chilly. I would hate to have the radiation gun overheat! No *Star Trek* phasers on overload needed here!

They had a mask that had been custom-made for me that I saw for the first time, and that couldn't be worn over clothing. It went from my shoulder region up over my head and made with a see-through mesh, so I wasn't blind. It looked like something medieval-jousting knights might wear, if it were made of metal. On it, they had marked specific places where they wanted to target the radiation beam, and when I was settled on a table, they would work on each side of me, aligning it just right. Then they asked if I could hear the music okay, and then skedaddled out of the room, closing a large vault-like door to the outside. Clang!

The treatment consisted of the Intensity Modulated Radiation Therapy (IMRT) technique. This is a computer-controlled approach that used precise targeting of the tumor based on a 3-D model created from my previous CT-Scan and MRI review. It "sculpted" around the tumor so that surrounding tissue would be less affected. While in the radiation chamber, I could hear the device rotating around me, shooting the radiation in at various strengths based on the target it was shooting at. Kind of like different calibers of bullets could be loaded into the same gun, based on what they had to go through, plastic, wood, car windshields, concrete, etc. No "Smart Gun" exists like this now; I'm sure it would be handy to prevent collateral damage. I remember someone advising to watch out for the caliber gun you bought for home defense. You wouldn't necessarily want a shotgun if you lived in a crowded apartment complex for fear of the shot tearing through the walls into the apartments next to you! This computer-controlled radiation gun technique, IMRT, tried to avoid collateral damage as much as possible.

The actual radiation treatment would last for about ten minutes long, taking twenty minutes total including doing a visual ID and dressing, etc. They let me bring in my own CDs and also had Pandora available if I just wanted to listen to any particular genre of music like alternative, Motown, or '80s rock. They had a computer screen with my picture and vitals on it and every time they asked, "Is this you?" These people were fun but not playing around with misidentifying anyone.

I like rock in all its styles. I brought in CDs by Yes (lots of longer tunes), some faster paced tunes by Prince and Led Zeppelin, a Motown classics CD with a lot of energy, and a great Genesis greatest hits CD that the hospital owned that we played, although I was bummed that we couldn't hear all of Suppers' Ready (twenty-three minutes). We split that one over two days. I even brought some Aaron Copeland in once when feeling a bit patriotic to hear Henry Fonda do the narration for the Lincoln portrait for President's Day. The staff were a little surprised, but I'd worked at a classical radio station in Denver and discovered the piece then. It fitted the treatment time perfectly and was inspiring to listen to. A guy can't be too predictable!

The actual treatment was painless, although it was really doing a number inside me. The music I picked was a great distraction for me. I learned that distraction from thinking about a bad thing with thinking about a good thing was a Jedi mind trick I could play on myself to control my own attitude. I thought that by not thinking about the actual treatment going on, the less stressed I was, and the more effective the treatment would be. Just having the belief that it would work, lying back, and enjoying the tunes had a healing outcome…kind of like what happened in my golf game! When I was finally able to play again that summer, I was so grateful to be able to play again that nothing bothered me, and I had some of the best rounds of my life!

4. Happy Birthday, Mom

January 25, 2018

Not feeling nearly as punked out as I did yesterday. I got a lot of sleep. I was feeling bad last night though so I called off going to my mother Eleanor's memorial birthday mass today. She wouldn't have wanted me struggling to get there, and Dad had masses scheduled for her, her parents, and my sister, Betty, almost every month this year.

Coincidentally this is also the feast day of the conversion of Saint Paul. His story forms the basis of one of my all-time-favorite books, *The Greatest Salesman in the World* by Og Mandino. Too many gems of wisdom to relate here, but the most apropos for this ugly week is "This too shall pass." Thanks to all for your support!

Comments:

Ray W.

Hang in there brother. You've got a big family caring about you. Missing loved one's on milestones is never easy. If you have their memory, you have them forever.

Cindy M.

Also, St. Julian of Norwich. "All shall be well, all shall be well and all manner of things shall be well."

Extended version:

This was the first week when the CaringBridge platform really kicked into gear, relaying news of my condition to many different groups of people in my life. My circles of friends, family, and work colleagues all learned about things and could respond just from one post by me.

Thanks to my chemo-brain though, I didn't notice how to respond. Once I saw how to make replies after a few more days of journal entries, I did feel like an idiot, kind of sheepish. I've always been good about technical things, but I think it was a combination of the drugs I had in my body and maybe pride I had about appearing stoic, that somehow prevented me from responding right away, individually. I was glad when I found out later how to do this though.

In reflection, all the positive CaringBridge comments really went a long way in helping me overcome cancer. In doing some brief research on the topic (There are hundreds of studies.), it seems optimism and resilience go hand in hand. Your endurance or your resilience to sickness is not just controlled by the steroids or antibiotics being pumped into you but by the dopamine and endorphins released inside you by all the love and support expressed in those comments. So if you get sick and require long term treatment, use those social platforms you have and combine them into one BIG CaringBridge audience for the duration of your struggle.

As you can tell, going to mass plays a big part in my family's life. I was brought up Roman Catholic, was an altar boy in grade school, and as life has progressed and I traveled around the country, I always sought out a local church to belong to. My mom had actually gone into a convent after high school but decided the life wasn't for her, although she maintained her strong faith all through her life. She needed that, especially being married to a Cleveland police officer who had a very tough, dangerous job. She fell ill and passed away quickly on January 5, 2017, less than a year before my sister and I got sick. We'd always been trying to go with my dad; I even officially switched parishes so I'd get collection envelopes from where I was attending, Mary Queen of the Apostles. After Betty fell ill it was just me and my brother going with Dad that fall.

Needless to say, not being able to go to weekly masses was missed. Everyone knew my immune system was compromised; the doctor had even charted out which days between chemo treatments how vulnerable I'd be. Looked like a stock market chart—high, then gradually plunging, then a slow recovery. But I digress.

Somehow, I can't remember (thanks chemo brain), I received a copy of a monthly publication called *The Word Among Us*. It's a daily review of mass readings and meditations on the Scripture readings. Great for shut-ins like me! I couldn't have communion but could read and reflect each day on what would be said in that specific day's mass, for instance, today's reading being the feast day of Saint Paul.

A life-long favorite book of mine is Og Mandino's *The Greatest Salesman in the World*. Whether or not sales is your profession, it's a great book on the human condition. We all deal with people, even shut-ins! The book is practical as well as spiritual and a fast read! It is formatted into very small chapters (handy when fatigued) that included this famous quote, "This too will pass." I reminded myself of it many times.

I learned about it from a guy I hired for the telephone-solicitation room I managed while working for Preview-Subscription TV in 1981 before cable came into Cleveland. We sold a single, scrambled signal that carried uncut, commercial-free movies, sports events, concerts, and soft-core comedic porn late at night—a little bush and boobies, nothing serious, but a lot of guys bought the service just for that. Anyway, Bill was a retiree from AT&T who started his career selling telegraph services! He thought this would be fun, and in our interview he mentioned this book to me, which I followed up on and eventually passed around the staff. Later on, I was hired as an installation specialist, who'd be travelling around the country installing software for broadcasting station operations, and guess what type of training I had? Yep, besides the technical stuff we all had to take "Psychology of Selling" to polish our human relation skills.

Og Mandino's book covers the story of a camel boy who made good the birth of Christ and the trials of St. Paul, a persecutor of

Christ's disciples in the early years of Christianity. He had a miraculous conversion and tried to preach, but no one would trust him or listen to what he had to say. He's told in a vision to seek out the ex-camel boy and learn from him. To make a long story short, he received ten scrolls that detail what you need to be a success. They are the following:

1. Begin a new life with good habits
2. The importance of love
3. The power of persistence
4. You are nature's greatest miracle
5. Live this day like it's your last
6. Master your emotions with positive action
7. Laugh at the world
8. Multiply your value with goals
9. Act now
10. Pray

These are all-powerful life lessons; each scroll takes about five minutes to read. Whether you're a cancer patient, caregiver, recovering addict, or an injured athlete, this book will build up your faith, optimism, and resilience to overcome whatever challenges you face.

5. Bye bye Taste Buds

January 28, 2018

One week down! Yay!

The good news is the side effects from chemo went by quickly; I did a lot of hydration trying to get that poison out of my system. Bad news is that taste over the weekend really went away from the daily radiation faster than I thought. I have been hydrating, doing mouthwashes, etc. but still could not taste a burger last night and a lot of other stuff since. I still have some tasty dishes that Kathy made too, dagnabit. They'll come back though, just have to power through this phase until summer or so. Like a nurse once told me I'll learn to appreciate the consistency of things, which I am, like w/ guacamole!

I got caught up on my scripture readings today 'cause I opted out of mass. Too much sickness around and this second week I'm in the "nadir" phase of chemo, low resistance for seven to fourteen days out from first chemo hit. I will have to miss OLA's first Friday services too. Bummer! Plan to be a hermit this week outside of radiation visits.

Friday was the feast day of Saints Timothy and Titus. One passage from the daily mass was from the first reading, Second Timothy and some bracing advice from Saint Paul "For God did not give us a spirit of cowardice but rather of power and love and self-control."

Listening to not exactly church music but some relaxing Tubular Bells.

Thanks to all for your comforting messages and support. Will catch up w/ you soon!

Comments:

Lisa R.

You got this Ed! Hang in there, we are all pulling for you!

Pattie M.

God Bless You!!! Prayers

Pam T.

Hang in there Ed! Those taste buds will return!

Extended version:

I'm a Libra, so I like balancing the bad news with the good whenever possible. After just five radiation treatments, it seemed my saliva glands and taste buds were getting pretty damaged. I used some of the national brands for preventing dry mouth the radiology team gave me. I had never noticed the TV commercials before, but now I see them all the time!

One of my sister's hospice nurses had told me the line about enjoying the consistency of things like guacamole. In these early stages, don't expect that appreciation to kick in yet. In fact, expect a little anger, denial, and general grouchiness over the gradual decline of taste. And it's not that the taste buds are "gone," and you don't taste anything…what you taste tastes like crap. So the consistency of guacamole gives as much enjoyment as munching on chips and mud.

Verse was from 2 Timothy 1:7, and in my present state of mind at that point, was appreciated. I was missing first Friday services for Our Lady of Angels, under kind of a self-imposed house arrest based on what I learned in chemo class and rapidly not being able to enjoy my favorite foods, not to mention no alcohol. First Friday "services" was actually a get together of mostly guys who went to school at OLA to drink, reminisce, plan golf outings, and basically catch up on things. We rotate through neighborhood bars of which in a mostly Irish-German neighborhood, there are a lot. These friends did give me a lot of support once word was passed that I was sick. I would've liked to have seen them but knew it'd be for the best if I skipped it. I shunned being a buzz-killer.

As the verse says, God gave us all a spirit of power and love and self-control. Yes, I had to stay out from enjoying fun social events. Yes, I had to eat bad-tasting food as long as I could before the throat became too raw. But these conditions needed to be overcome, not with self-pity or paranoia but by the grace of God and the Holy Spirit, not to become bitter but to keep an optimistic, strong frame of mind.

> *"You aren't going to find anybody that's going to be successful without making a sacrifice and without perseverance"* (Lou Holtz).

Oddly enough, the long twenty-four-minute video piece I shared was "Tubular Bells" by Mike Oldfield, the theme from the movie, *The Exorcist*. In hindsight, perfectly apropos as I was undergoing treatment to exorcise the cancer out of my body! And like I would discover, the treatment started softly but in a creepy way, picked up in violent intensity, broke off into syncopated multi-instrument riffs (like the various elements of treatment: chemo, radiation, calories and hydration, all in measured amounts), then became joyous, and finally mellowed out to a simple, peaceful finish, a soundtrack for more than a movie but for my ordeal in trying to get well!

6. Just a Month Ago

January 30, 2018

It's hard to believe my sister, Betty, just passed on December 30, 2017. It seems like forever. I miss you, B!

Comments:

Patricia H.

Ed, praying that your treatments are going well. We serve an awesome God that LOVES ALL HIS CHILDREN. Keep up the FAITH and HE will never leave you nor forsake you. Blessings. Pat.

Extended version:

There is a picture of me when I had Tom text Betty after I had my neck tumor biopsy on November 30. I was hoping they got everything in one fell swoop with the blade, but a few weeks later I was told that was not the case. The biopsy indicated stage 4B oropharyngeal cancer. Stage 4C would've been terminal so I had a fighting chance. Betty, on the other hand, had an inoperable brain tumor that could not be treated with radiation and chemotherapy.

7. Two Weeks Down, Five to Go

February 2, 2018

R adiation treatments have been going by quick, especially since I've been bringing in prog rock CDs from Genesis, and Yes, they have more than nine minute tunes, about the length of time I stay in the machine.

Tasting less and less, and what I taste is usually not good; but like I told my dad, guys—in WWII and Korea War and other wars—had to eat s— on a shingle for months. I can handle doing that for a while, just have to remind myself NOT to avoid eating, keep my strength up, and always brush afterward because salivary glands are "out to lunch." Pardon the pun.

Binged watching *Blacklist* TV series and just picked up *Artemis* by Andy Weir, author of *The Martian*.

I have signed up for LinkedIn Sales Navigator and have found it's very effective. I improved my profile with eight professional trade reviews of 40+ New Revenue Sources and network jumped over fifty this week to eight hundred plus

Really trying to avoid chemo brain and the pull of the couch for naps. I missed Blues Traveler in Cleveland this week. I have seen them before, and they're a great high-energy harmonica—based band. This funny video talks a bit about cancer and has Woody Harrelson in freaky snippets from the film *Kingpin*.

"Someday an answer will find us, quite a long shot,
But anyway, I think the past the past is behind us.
Be real confusing if not but anyway
I put all my hope in tomorrow, it's gonna be great.
I can tell but anyway I see a new, a new day dawning.
I like to sleep late, oh well, but anyway."

Blues Traveler, But Anyway

Comments:

Dave M.

Love old Genesis, especially Super's Ready. You rock Ed. You have a great attitude. Dave

Fern B.

Keep the faith, that's what it's all about. Thinking and praying.

Extended version:

I always liked progressive rock when growing up in the mid '70s. I played the triple album *Yessongs* stacked up on my record player over and over, never dreamed then how useful they'd be in a radiation room. But the songs "Heart of the Sunrise," "Yours is No Disgrace," "Starship Trooper," and many others helped take my mind off things and being eight to ten minutes in length were great for the short bursts I had to go through for five days a week. Likewise I listened to the whole *Lamb Lies Down on Broadway* double album CD, plus *Watcher of the Skies*, *Firth of Fifth*, *Musical Box*, and many others on a great compilations CD the radiology team had in their room.

As I remember from old health classes in school, the tongue has taste buds that detect four main flavors: salty, sweet, bitter, and sour. As I understand it, saliva carries food molecules when we eat to get absorbed by these various buds. Radiation treatment (for my particular kind of throat cancer) could not avoid blasting through the area where the salivary glands and taste buds are. And I was discovering, the last of the buds to survive must've been the bitter ones. They say after a nuclear war the last surviving animals will be cockroaches. Well, the bitter buds must be the cockroaches of the tongue.

Once upon a time in my mid twenties, my go to drink was rum and Coke. Free Cuba, order me a Cuba Libre, yay! Then a daughter in the house I was rooming at when I lived in Connecticut was dating a dentist, and on learning I hadn't visited a dentist in two years because of my new job in a new state, suggested I visit him. He discovered a gold mine in my mouth from all the cavities. He used tough love, showing me with a mirror all the holes he drilled out that he had to fix. Needless to say, afterward I quit the sugary drinks and started religiously brushing my teeth. No more cavities for close to forty years! However, on learning what was happening with the radiation and salivary glands, I made sure to brush five times a day, after meals and before and after hitting the sack. It must've worked because that summer nothing was wrong with the teeth. These treatments could've caused me to get them all extracted and wear dentures! I hate drilling, and the prospects of dentures really made me feel old! I have enough problems with this, I don't need any more!

I thought I'd be lounging around watching TV and reading, but that was not the case. I was getting fatigued from not sleeping for more than a few hours at a stretch and not eating right. Most two-hour movies took me two days to finish; I rarely watched more than one episode at a time of *Blacklist* (although it's a great show), and reading more than four pages would cause me to wake up forty-five minutes later with a sore back and dry eyes.

Man does not live by vitamin pills and placid behavior alone. Focusing on a future after cancer can help cure you as well. I chose to start building up a network of contacts for LinkedIn to help spread the word about my book, *40+ New Revenue Sources for Libraries and Nonprofits*. I would zone out even doing this for forty-five minutes. However, despite the fatigue, planning and working toward the future by setting my goals for book contacts helped with my overall attitude. Working on my part-time entrepreneurial project had helped make me a little money but more importantly would be helpful for people struggling to improve or keep open their library or nonprofit, and was fun. And to paraphrase what Sergeant Horvath says in *Saving Private Ryan*, "Maybe doing something good in the middle of this whole god-awful shitty mess" will earn me the right to live.

If you can, check out the video with Blues Traveler and Woody Harrelson. I never did rent the movie, but it's a high-energy song with some funny moments and some gross scenes around a toilet I thought I would shortly be relating to. In my current condition the phrase, "But anyway," definitely fit. You can tell about your pain and discomfort to people, then spin it by saying, "But anyway." That helps release the pressure and pain by keeping you focused on the future. Despite all that, recognizing the past, the cancer, whatever the current SH—T on a shingle is in your life, say "But anyway, I'm gonna think this, see this, hope this, do this…"

> "*Earn the right to be proud and confident*" (John Wooden).

8. Timely Feast Day!

February 4, 2018

This weekend the church observes the feast day of Saint Blaise with the blessing of throats. He was a premedieval bishop and doctor, who was martyred by being beaten, attacked with iron combs (don't even want to research those!), then beheaded. Then the first reading was from the Old Testament Book of Job, "*I have been assigned months of misery.*" Cheery.

But both men kept the faith and that helped them remain relevant centuries later. Pastor's message today broke down their lessons into three things we can all practice: word, action, and prayer. That is, expressing ourselves to each other honestly, taking action when needed, and communicating with the Almighty in whatever way we are most comfortable with. Good thoughts to start week three!

Throat condition from radiation is getting a bit more painful, and taste, as opposed to being gone, is still there. Just everything tasting oily or bitter. I joked with the pastor in the vestibule after services that I was going to lift my shirt and have him bless my PEG tube, my alternate throat in probably two more weeks. He laughed, said no. Blessing is a one size fits all type of thing, covers the whole body!

Go, Eagles!

Comments:

Simone N.

Keeping you in my prayers. Miss seeing you at Woods, but think of you often. Glad things are going well so far, but sorry to hear about the taste issue. I know how bad that can be. This will be over soon enough and then we will have a party at Woods! Stay strong and keep smiling :)

Patricia P.
Ed,

Enjoyed your note and sense of humor! Glad to see that even in this difficult time you can keep the amazing sense of humor. I am sure it helps you get through difficult days. Sending loving thoughts and prayers your way...your Georgia family!

Extended version:

The quote is from Job 7:3, and I didn't get it exactly right in writing in my CaringBridge journal entry. The closest I can find now is the New Living translation: "*I too have been assigned months of futility, long, and weary nights of misery.*" These would definitely come in time.

This was one of my principal reasons for fatigue, lack of proper sleep. I went to a "Science Café" once about sleep. These are usually hosted in bars of craft brewery where you can catch a buzz and maybe learn a thing or two about some cool subject. A fun-early-date activity makes her think you are smart. There I remember learning about sleep cycles that last for ninety minutes, and ideally you should have four to six per night. Even after a year since I finished treatments, I still frequently wake up with dry mouth at all times of the night. What I try to do is catch at least ninety minutes of sleep sometime. Generally, if I set an alarm these days at seven and have been up three to four times at night, knowing I didn't get a full uninterrupted ninety minutes, I reset the alarm for maybe one hundred more minutes. I have what I call "sleep traction" in the morning. If I wake up tired and there are no pressing concerns, it's easier for me to fall and stay asleep for one extra cycle than any other time of the day. More sleep equals more energy to get well.

Job went through many trials as does every cancer patient. The reference to the Eagles was about my high school mascot. My high school was then going into the 2018 regional basketball playoffs. Many of my CaringBridge followers were also either guys from Saint Edward High School in Lakewood, Ohio, or knew of my attachment to them. The school and especially the football program that I was a part of was great in teaching me the discipline for both strength building and conservation. We took salt pills all the time during a two-a-day August drills, drank piss warm Gatorade, clustered under the few trees around our practice field to catch shade during short rest periods. These physical survival actions, even though I went through them over forty years before, stuck with me as I entered what was essentially the only other physical survival battle I'd have over my sixty-one years of age.

Saint Edward's was good for laying down the basics of physical and spiritual endurance. Taking advantage of the lessons from the coaches and the blessings of Saint Blaise definitely helped pull me through.

A friend of mine, Rosemary, after reading this entry, sent me a prayer card from another saint. This one is targeted toward cancer. Saint Peregrine had a vision of Christ coming down from the cross to heal him of his cancer. He is the patron saint of those with cancer and has a prayer that helped me focus my wishes for healing for myself and others:

> "Saint Peregrine, you are honored as the patron of all cancers. You are known as the miracle worker. You suffered from cancer and with your strong devotion to God, were cured. Deliver me from the cancer that afflicts my body. I ask for your most needed intervention before God to save me and cure me so I may live to spread God's glory. If needed, I ask, O glorious saint, for a miracle. Pray for me."

9. Transitioning Tastes

February 8, 2018

Never thought I'd say this but I'm glad I'm starting to lose taste. Since last week, most things tasted really bad. Now I just can't taste them. Today I tried meatballs, shrimp, and fajita chicken strips. The shrimp was tasteless but went down okay. The other two dried out in my mouth immediately but went down okay w/ sips of water. I can live w/ that. Kathy and I met w/ speech therapist who reviewed what happens w/ the throat tissue during these radiation treatments and gave me some good advice and exercises to do in a "worst case scenario" if I'm not eating or talking much for weeks at a time. I am in the third week of seven, ugh. Good to be prepared though. Southwest General Health Center really covers the bases!

Today is the feast day of Saint Jerome Emiliani. The following quote from him is inspiring, especially if you exchange the word fire with radiation:

"God wishes to test you like gold in the furnace. The dross is consumed by the fire, but the pure gold remains and its value increases."

Radiation is tough but necessary. My cancer cells are getting zapped!

Check out this violent, aggressive video by AC/DC to catch my drift…Thunderstruck

Very motivating! Almost makes me want to go twice a day… almost.

Thunder!

AC/DC, Military Montage to the song Thunderstruck

Comments:

Margie R.

Keep STRONG Brother—Rock it OUT

Larry S.

Excellent video. Great motivation. Keep the faith Ed.

Extended version:

The *Military Montage* was a great series of film clips of the following military vehicles firing their guns or dropping bombs that exploded in perfect synchronization to the rhythms of Thunderstruck: an AC-130, F-35, A-10, M1 Abrams, B-2, AH-64 Apache Longbow, USS Missouri BB-63, F/A-18, and a F-117. What guy doesn't like ship cannons, tanks, helicopters, and jets firing missiles in sync with heavy metal music? It also feels good watching it because of the mental cathartic release that it brings. I can't see what the radiation is doing to the cancer cells. I can "feel the burn" as the taste buds and salivary glands are being destroyed and can only hope that the little cancer buggers are being blasted to hell like the targets in the video. That would make the sacrificing of enjoying food and drink worth it!

A fellow librarian friend, Audrey, commented after watching the video (the first time she saw an AC/DC video I'm sure) "Oh, Ed, you're such a *guy*!" hence, the inspiration for my title!

I was surprised when a speech therapist showed up after my treatment today. She gave me some sheets with exercises and tongue twisters. I majored in communications at Cleveland State University and took a speech class there that changed my life. It taught me different breathing techniques and how to project my voice differently. Shortly after I started my broadcasting career at the campus radio station and found I could fire off long descriptions of songs without going "uh…" several times in a sentence. Ever since those days I've always felt good about tongue twisters and make it a point to look (or hear) for them in everyday situations and to say to anyone close by, "Try to say that five times fast." Try it with that last phrase I used in quotes. So I thought I knew everything. Wrong!

> "*A man's pride can be his downfall, and he needs to learn when to turn to others for support and guidance*" (Bear Grylls).

The therapist gave me sheets with a number of laryngeal and base of tongue exercises like pretending to gargle without water, speech exercises for the back of the tongue like saying "sing, sang, song, sung," and prolonging the "ng" sound for five seconds, the "masako maneuver" sticking your tongue out and trying to swallow, fun stuff like that and jaw-opening exercises. She also gave me nutrient dense soft food recipes. My favorite was the banana-protein milkshake. I still have two to three of these a week and have added peanut powder to it. I used peanut butter at first, but that made things sticky in my blender, making it a pain to clean.

> "*I've been blessed to find people who are smarter than I am, and they help me to execute the vision I have*" (Russell Simmons).

The speech therapist like the other people in my treatment plan, the radiation and infusion center teams, the nutritionists, and of course, my radiologist, oncologist, and ear, nose, and throat doctors were great and very thorough in making sure I understood what was going on with me. I sent them all Christmas cards, telling them I counted them as among my blessings in this past tough year of 2018.

10. Hello, Old Friends

February 12, 2018

I had my second chemo treatment today, one more to go in three weeks. I am pumped up on steroids now; the next few days will be different, not *difficult,* in my frame of mind. Whatever situation I find myself in, I try to keep that attitude. Whether the issue is money, work, romance, grief, or sickness, being different is a short-term solution-oriented outlook, IMHO. Difficult is a downer, no win, no end in sight.

Perhaps I'm biased by today's first reading from First James. Shout out to cousin Jim in Brooklyn and my late Uncle Jim, who I did not meet enough times in this life, but gave me a lot of insights on how smart and tough my dad is.

> *"Consider it all joy, my brothers and sisters, when you*
> *encounter various trials, for you know that the testing*
> *of your faith produces perseverance"* (James 1:2–3).

I had three good buddies who connected with me this weekend. Phil sent me an "Irish package" from Colorado with music, jokes, and a great book *How the Irish Saved Civilization,* which I read years ago at the library, but now I have my own copy…sweet. Ben whom I haven't seen since we went to see a Genesis cover band a few years ago, and Art whom I just see three to four times a year, called from the "Merry Arts" in Lakewood. Ben lives in Arizona now, and he and his Peruvian wife Yrma stopped by Sunday to drop off some of the Peruvian free trade coffee they sell. Ben's been playing guitar for forty years. I remember him when he was first starting to play guitar. He has been trying to boost the local music scene in the Kingman, Arizona area and has written eighty songs. This goes out to him and all you others calling, sending cards and prayers my way. Hello, old friends!

> Hello, old friend!
> (Hello, old friend!)
> Really good to see you once again.
> > Eric Clapton, Hello Old Friend

Comments:

Pattie S.

Thanks for introducing me to that Eric Clapton song! Rock on!

Sal D.

Awesome, Ed!

Extended version:

Seeing I had a lot of friends and family keeping in contact with me on this platform, I couldn't help but give a shout out to those family members that I love called James. Especially given the fact that today's Scripture reading was from James. He used a "family" reference in his words on faith, creating perseverance. Yes, I was going through various trials, and both faith and friends gave me strength.

My chemo treatment always included steroids, which always gave me a strong boost for a couple of days before any bad symptoms occurred. Was the Scripture reading just a coincidence or a sign from my departed, Uncle Jimmy, to prepare myself? I think when you're in a battle like this, you need to be aware and draw strength from every source that you can. Your faith, loving friends, music, and "coincidental" events can build up inside you and create an attitude to either make you sick or well.

At this point, I had decided to not waste energy on self-pity. I began to despise the word "difficult," and would swap it whenever possible with "different." And whenever my supportive peeps would call and say they were supporting me through this difficult time with various prayers and actions, I tried to spin it that things at this time were just different. Healthy or sick, our condition in this life is always changing, and for me now, it was just 'different.' That attitude helped me persevere. "Different, not difficult"…I might make that into a T-Shirt slogan!

That and gestures from friends had really helped me pull through, like Art telling me he was getting two tix for a David Byrne concert that is coming to Cleveland this summer. We went to see him in the '90s together (with complimentary tickets from the radio station I worked at). He wanted to do a payback. I was not talking well, and I was staying inside to avoid catching anything in my weakened state. But I let him know I'd be better and there with him in six months (which I was). Phil, Ben, and I hadn't seen each other in years due to distance, but we kept in touch. Thanks to the internet.

Pharmaceuticals may help cure, but people help you heal.

11. Hump Day

February 14, 2018

The feast of Ash Wednesday was today. I am ashamed to say I was too beat to get any but read through the Mass readings for today, "Remember that you are dust, and to dust you shall return." And Happy Valentine's Day to all of you who show your love daily to the sick, the young, and each other. It's also Hump Day for my treatments! Three-and-a-half weeks out of seven for radiation, I had the second of three chemo treatments on Monday. Nausea and fatigue gradually dissipating.

Peter Gabriel's "San Jacinto" to me touches on healing in the Native American way: sweat lodges, medicine men, rattlesnake bites. Toughness and tenacity. Good imagery too. Enjoy!

> I hold the line, the line of strength that pulls me
> through the fear
> San Jacinto, I hold the line
> San Jacinto, the poison bite and darkness take
> my sight, I hold the line
> And the tears roll down my swollen cheek, think
> I'm losing it, getting weaker
> I hold the line, I hold the line.
>
> Peter Gabriel, San Jacinto

Comments:

Charles B.

Glad to hear of your progress. Your faith and tenacity will get you though this!

Cindy M.

Remember that you are dust that matters to God! And to your friends and coworkers! When you've finished your treatments and are feeling a little stronger, if you want to participate in a sweat lodge, I can hook you up with one at the Ursuline Motherhouse.

Extended version:

Ashes and Indians, today both cultures merged for me. The ashes from the various Bible readings in Genesis and Ecclesiastes that remind us of our mortality. The Indian culture from the readings by one of my favorite authors, Carlos Casteneda, who chronicled the philosophy of a southwestern Yaqui Indian "man of knowledge," Don Juan, and a great song about an Apache ceremony by Peter Gabriel.

Castaneda became popular in the sixties by doing his PhD dissertation about Don Juan and his use of peyote to enter into altered states. I discovered him in college through friends as we passed around (among other things) Casteneda's books, as well as writers like Tom Wolfe, author of *The Electric Kool-Aid Acid Test*, and Hunter S. Thompson's *Fear and Loathing in Las Vegas*.

But a larger part of Casteneda's books did not deal with peyote at all, in fact, Don Juan said they were a necessary evil and should be stopped at a certain point. Most of the books concern the warrior's lifestyle ("only a warrior can one withstand the path of knowledge" from *Tales of Power*), which among its many rules was "using death as an advisor." Like in the Christian celebration of Ash Wednesday, the acknowledgment of death is a reminder that we have only a little amount of time on this earth. Don't use it whining or complaining. Take things as a challenge, and if things seem really, really bad (like they do a few days after chemo), check in with your death. Death, according to Don Juan, is always just a few feet away in your left. If you see a shadow or something weird, it's just your death, like a guardian angel letting you know he hasn't touched you yet. It helps make you humble and not as concerned with just a little paltry puking.

The music video shows a variety of Native American oriented paintings in fantastic colors. It also includes some photography from the 1800s and cool picture of Mount Rushmore with four photos of Indian leaders like Geronimo and Sitting Bull above them. The lyrics came from Peter Gabriel's conversation with an Apache Indian about rite of passage in becoming a Brave when he was fourteen that all young men went through. He told of a hike up a mountain with a medicine man that called for being bitten by a rattlesnake (instead of using peyote). The challenge was then being left on a mountain, and they either make their way down or die.

The narrator in the song has fever-inspired visions, seeing below the land as the white man will make it, describing the clash of cultures. The lyric, "hold the line," to me, describes the tenacity of the Brave going through the ceremony, as well as the struggle to keep his native culture alive. "Hold the line" becomes a chant in the end, invoking the survival that will happen if you just hang in there, if you just hold the line and keep moving.

According to an internet review of the song on songfacts.com and the conversation he had with the Apache, "this story got Gabriel thinking about how many cultures had rituals where young men are forced to face death, which can teach courage and foster an appreciation for life." Much like the Christian ritual of Ash Wednesday. Who knew we had that in common with the Apaches! We are all part of the same universe, created by God.

"Every day is a gift from God. There's no guarantee of tomorrow, so that tells me to see the good in this day to make the most of it" (Joel Osteen).

I thought of how apropos that Lent was beginning on Ash Wednesday, just as I was beginning the second half of the treatments. I mentioned that the effects from chemo that week were dissipating just to make my friends and family a little more at ease. I didn't give up anything specifically for Lent like we did as kids, giving up chocolate or something else we liked as a form of repentance for Jesus's upcoming sacrifice for us. But I did decide to downplay the chemo effects in my CaringBridge comments. People who actually saw me could see the effects. The second chemo round was much tougher than the first to recover from, and the third would be tougher yet. The CaringBridge comments were all great though. The one above about the local Cleveland sweat lodge was from my boss, Cindy, who also turned me onto CaringBridge. Those comments and support really helped me "hold the line."

12. Yum, Smoothies!

February 18, 2018

Just a bit of sarcasm there. I'm on full liquid diet now through the PEG tube, which, of course, I can't taste, but if I have any leftover after this, I can make it into smoothies. A good way to get two thousand calories and a lot of protein and other nutritious stuff into me.

So to celebrate, enjoy the "Smoothie Song" by Nickel Creek. Reminds me a little of Blues Brothers music store scene. Who hasn't seen that?

Comments:

Nicolette P.

I love Nickel Creek! We saw them live in Cleveland years ago. Glad you have so much good music to accompany you on your journey since you can't have comfort food right now. Your fan club is pulling for you, Ed!

Tom R.

Stay Strong Bro—3 weeks to go!

Extended version:

About one month after radiation treatments started, my throat was so burned that I started using my food tube full time (formally called a percutaneous endoscopic gastrostomy or PEG tube). I had it inserted into my stomach around January 17, keeping it secured through tape to my chest to move around easier. It was a necessary evil, and I still can't believe my second-opinion doctor said a PEG tube was one part of the treatment he would not do…unless I was really hurting. Damn! When I was really hurting, I would not have wanted the PEG surgery and complications that operation could've caused during my chemo and radiation periods.

Made to deliver a thick liquid that was "calorically dense, complete nutrition with fiber," it contained 375 calories, 17 grams of protein, 44 carbs, and a lot of vitamins. I was also given a pill crusher, and when I wasn't using the tube for taking nutrition, I'd crush vitamins, pain-killers, and poop pills, mix them with water and down them that way. They gave me a goal of sixty-four ounces of hydration to do each day.

It extended out about eight inches, and I used a funnel to pour a carton, 8.45 fluid ounces of liquid nutrition down the tube easier. My fluid was created by Nestlé, the chocolate syrup maker, which prompted fond memories of making chocolate milk as a kid. Believe it or not, as an adult, this was much more messy! I always had a towel in my lap because holding the carton in one hand and coordinating the funnel into the tube always caused a little spillage, until doing it for a few weeks. I used medical tape to secure the tube without the funnel back to my chest when finished. It never occurred to me to use tape on the funnel to keep it in place when I was doing it my myself. Next time… which I hope never happens again! I used that funnel prior to being sick to pour Crown Royal, Jameson, and other liquid refreshments into flasks for golf. Looking forward to using it again for that someday.

Regarding the challenges of swallowing, I was able to do Nyquil when I was sick with the flu the following winter after treatments, which burned but did the trick. From there, I progressed to Jägermeister. Soon maybe, stronger "medicine." Beer has also been a measure of progress. Two months after losing the food tube, I couldn't have Bud Light or any domestic beer; the carbonation really hurt my throat. Then a friend of mine, Pat, a home brewer, suggested I try IPAs. Lo and behold, those went down much better! Then Guinness Stout soon after, and that was good. Eight months after treatment, and I'm back to non-fancy beers like Bud Light, my favorite. Yes, although there was a minor dark period when going full-time on the food tube, thinking I would never eat or drink normally again, I found that over time there is a Bud Light at the end of the tunnel!

I'm now using the leftover "calorically dense" liquid nutrition cartons to make my own smoothies with peanut butter powder, bananas, and other frozen fruit. Have tried chocolate syrup, but that addition tastes "different" for now. This too will pass!

"And St. Francis said: *'My dear son, be patient, because the weaknesses of the body are given to us in this world by God for the salvation of the soul. So they are of great merit when they are borne patiently'*" (St. Francis of Assisi).

The video has no lyrics but shows the band walking into a really cool musical instrument store (check out the guitar stems used as rails on the front door), picking up a few instruments, and doing an impromptu jam with another shopper, who was testing a stand-up bass, Rob Trujillo from Metallica! I'm lucky to live in Cleveland, home to many jam nights with excellent musicians appearing, several close to my home in the West Park neighborhood at bars named Kelleys, Smedley's, PJ McIntyre's and the Public House. It's great seeing impromptu team efforts. Team collaboration really helped with the food tube too. It was so much easier when my girlfriend, Kathy, helped pour as I held the tube and funnel steady.

The tube was a necessary evil, like so many other personal inconveniences that cancer causes. A card Kathy gave me paraphrased the following quote from Kay Yow, the legendary North Carolina's Women's basketball coach who had over 700 wins and now has a Cancer fund named in her honor. It frames the attitude you need to develop, one I'm sure she installed in all her players.

"When life kicks you, let it kick you forward" (Kay Yow).

13. The Waiting

February 25, 2018

Just two more weeks of treatments to go then a few more weeks for recovery! Each treatment week has had its own new challenges, but at least I can see light at the end of the tunnel. Thanks for all the calls, cards, and emails. Had a big card come in yesterday with a mockingjay seal on it, a resistance emblem from "*The Hunger Games,*" so I knew it had to be from a librarian. Fifteen of them actually. Thanks, team! Very inspiring in my fight. Just a few more weeks to wait and like the song says, "The waiting is the hardest part. Every day you see one more card. You take it on faith, you take it to the heart. The waiting is the hardest part..." Tom Petty and the Heartbreakers, The Waiting.

This 1981 video is pretty funny; I like the way they weren't taking it too seriously. Tom Petty was one of the most gifted musicians in my generation, amazing that he could smile and sing at the same time.

Comments:

Tonya E.

Hi Ed! I'm glad to see that the light at the end of the tunnel is appearing!

Mary O.

Hi Ed! You are a champ…always thinking of others and bolstering everybody. Well, you are always in my thoughts and I am sending healing wishes your way!

Extended version:

Tom Petty did this video when I was twenty-five, and he was thirty-one and just getting into the stride of his game. Decades would follow with a lot of great songs, but at the time, he did what he had to do, including making corny videos. I remember digging them though, even if the lip-synching was a little out of sync. I didn't realize the importance the lyrics would have for me back when I was twenty-five and feeling immortal.

In my battle with cancer, I was fairly isolated. I lived by myself, and although friends and family were nearby, outside of being given rides to daily radiation treatments, I spent a lot of time alone mostly because it was winter. There was the typical fear of the flu that was going around, and we were all concerned about them passing germs along to me. The chemo class in the beginning had really empha- sized sanitary protocols should be followed as much as possible. I suddenly had hand soap and antibacterial liquid in every room in my house. Thanks to the girls. The hospital seemed to have one out of every three people I saw wearing masks. When my sister, Betty, was battling her cancer in the fall, staff would come in and chastise us for not wearing them while visiting, so we all had the fear of God placed in us about being careful.

It was also strange for me not going to work, an environment where I'd come into contact with one hundred plus people a day, both patrons looking for help at the reference desk and my fellow staff. It wasn't like previous experiences away from work over the last twenty-five years when I'd enjoy traveling with friends and family to tourist spots or revisiting beautifully isolated spots in my old home of Colorado. I *was* able to enjoy the Jim Rome sports talk show, which came on my TV at noon each day; something I could never see while working, but the Jungle and talk radio really didn't count for interacting with real people.

Outside of listening to the Jungle (Rome's nickname for his call-in show environment), my human interaction was pretty low, and media really didn't count. That's why the CaringBridge platform came in handy; it was easy to have two-way exchanges! Other social media was okay; I'd never been into Facebook that much, always thought of it as too much of a time suck. Between my fatigue and lack of experience with that and Instagram, etc., CaringBridge made it so much easier reaching what is called in broadcasting my "core audience," people who were technically savvy and interested in my well-being. Between this new twenty-first-century tool and the old-style get-well cards that came in like Petty alluded to in his 1981 song, my isolation was pretty well chipped at. I still felt it but not as strong as it could've been.

Core audience is an important concept I believe in all aspects of your life: business, socially, in team sports—everything! Examples abound, like Arnie's Army, The Dawg Pound, Beatlemaniacs, Deadheads, Trekkies, the Twelfth Man, your Peeps. They are those who support you and give you momentum when you're weak, even if you don't want to admit it to yourself. While the clock kept ticking as this different time continued, and I waited on it to end, the cards and comments really helped. They say patience is a virtue. I'm not that virtuous, but the support from my core audience reminded me of Red Bull's slogan: it gave me wings!

14. Galvanize

February 28, 2018

Toughest week yet. I had painful constipation on Sunday, so I told radiation team on Monday, who said I'd done everything right, and blood tests from Friday showed I had low platelets and white blood cell count, so they sent me to the ER, where I had various tests and blood draws. Lots of docs involved. Also discovered I was possibly getting pneumonia. They kept me here and have been here at Southwest for three days. Pain is gone from Const. but still fatigued. They gave me iron and something to boost blood cells, as well as antibiotics and other stuff this afternoon. I had Kathy go to house to retrieve laptop and special food. Luckily Dad magically showed up and helped her out with stuff. Good signs like that keep happening, helping my spirits. That and the half-dozen Chemical Brothers working on me this week are helping me stay "Galvanized" against this mean ol' cancer.

> Put apprehension on the back burner, / let it sit, Don't even get it lit. Don't hold back! The world…(they're holding back…) The time has come to… The world…(you're holding back…) The time has come to… The world…(it's holding back…) The time has come to… To galvanize!
> The Chemical Brothers, Galvanize

Comments:

John H.

Your strength is amazing, fighting daily battles we are not aware of. Keep it up. I pray for you daily.

George B.

Day at a time, my good friend, a day at a time. We're thinking of you!!!

Extended version:

The song, "Galvanize," won a Grammy in 2006 for best dance recording. It shows three underage kids in clown paint, trying to sneak into a club to participate in krump dancing, a high energy form of dance from the street where people could unlock frustrated energy in a nonviolent way. Galvanize is a method of improving steel, and it also is used as a verb to "shock or excite someone to take action."

I really didn't want to complain about an embarrassing condition but did not want it to linger either. Constipation happens in a large part because of lack of hydration. Switching over to the food tube and not being very proficient with it yet alone, I fell behind on my own "watering" schedule and dried out my own insides. So despite only taking in liquid nutrition, no solids, I developed a massive bellyache that could not be relieved without help. I'll spare you the details but leave you with the warning…keep hydrated! Any great athlete can tell you that.

> *"As an athlete you've got to watch your hydration
> and your nutrition, and use the right kinds of fuel
> to help you perform your best"* (Derrick Brooks).

They did give me drugs after the last chemo treatment to alleviate this condition and advised MiraLax and milk of magnesia, neither of which worked. Without enough water, I guess these just got sucked up into my body before they could lubricate the parts you need to poop.

Between that and the low blood counts on some critical metrics, they decided to keep me in the hospital over the course of a few days and almost immediately thought I had pneumonia, which caused a few rounds of meds and X-rays. I had the same cute young girl for a hospital transport worker several times wheeling me through the hospital, which was fun and who was good at keeping my mind off what was a very annoying situation. The luck of the draw I guess!

Another blessing was having Kathy run to my house once I found out I'd be in the hospital a few days to get my laptop and a few other things. She arrived just at the same time Dad was dropping by to check my mail. He was able to help her with the equipment and find some books. Atheists would say lucky coincidence; believers like me say a blessing, thanks to Mom and Betty watching over my condition from heaven. Another sign saying our loved ones are never really gone, just out of sight for a while.

I guess I forgot to add a link to the song when I posted this entry to CaringBridge in my weakened state. It was in my head, but I forgot to activate the link. Thanks, chemo-brain! Luckily a librarian and colleague, Nicki, caught the fact I was missing my music and posted another video for me. A rollicking country tune that I was surprised she knew! Never judge a book by its cover, I guess. Rodney Atkins's "If You're Going Through Hell." He went to a school once to sing it for a girl with leukemia, according to a comment on the song's Youtube page. I loved it! A perfect song for fighting illness! Another blessing!

Comment:

Nicki P:

Drat. Mean Ol' Cancer, since you didn't post a song, I'll post one for you.

Rodney Atkins, If You're Goin' Through Hell

If you're goin' through hell keep on going / Don't slow down if you're scared don't show it / You might get out before the devil even knows you're there / When you're goin' through hell keep on movin' / Face that fire walk right through it / You might get out before the devil even knows you're there.

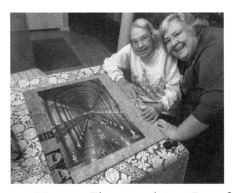

Puzzle Done—My mom Eleanor and sister Betty finishing a
puzzle of the library at Trinity College in Dublin.
I have this puzzle and picture hanging in my living room now.

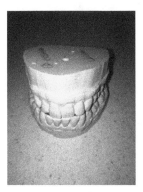

Teeth—Paperweights for my desk that
Stephen King would be proud of!

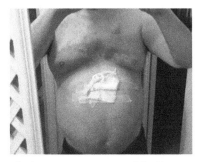

Peg tube—Prophylactic precautions. My Port in the upper-left
chest to avoid dozens of needles in my arm, and a food tube
for when I couldn't swallow food (or beer) anymore.

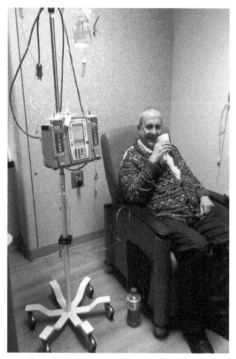

1st Chemo—Life is good! Enjoying the easy life in the easy chair.

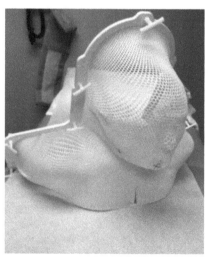

Mask—I should've kept this custom-made mask for
Halloween! The calibration marks were specific to targeting
my cancer region. Helped the team line things up perfectly.

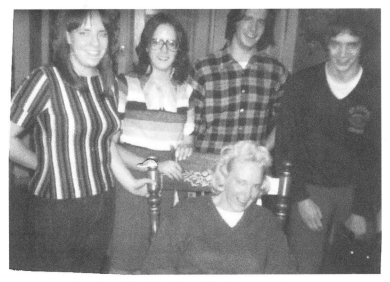

70s family—Wish Dad could've been in this picture,
but there were no such things as selfies in the seventies.
Betty, Annie, me in my Neil Young phase, brother
Tom, our dog Inky in the corner, and Mom.

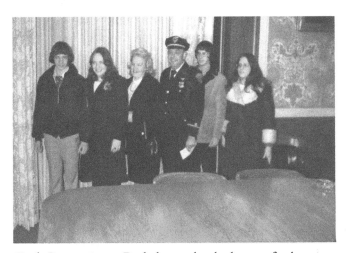

Dads Promotion—Dad always thanked mom for keeping
us under control when he studied for his promotional
exams! He became a sergeant in the late 60s. This was
for becoming captain in the late 70s. I was living out
of town when he became Deputy Chief in the 80s.

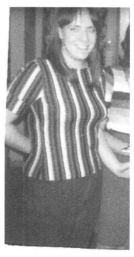

Betty 70s—One of the few pictures I had
on the Caring Bridge Platform.

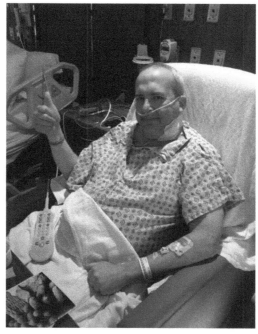

UH113017 After tumor removal—A picture I texted my sister
after I had my neck tumor removed, Nov. 30th, 2017. We were
both still optimistic about our conditions at that point.

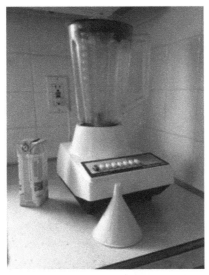

Blender—A funnel I used to fill whiskey flasks with that
I now used to get liquid nutrition into my narrow food
tube, until I could use and swallow blender drinks.

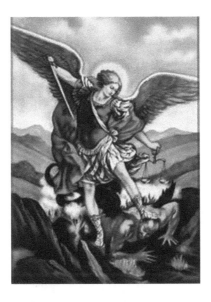

St. Michael—An inspiring picture. You have to weaponize
your personal activity to fight against cancer. Don't
depend on just radiation and chemotherapy.

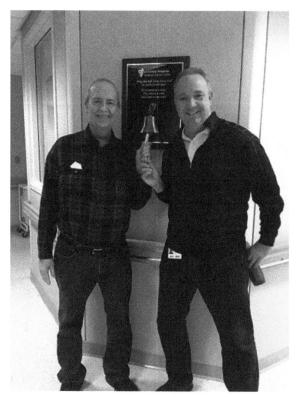

Bell and Bro's—Was fun for everyone ringing
the bell after the last radiation treatment!

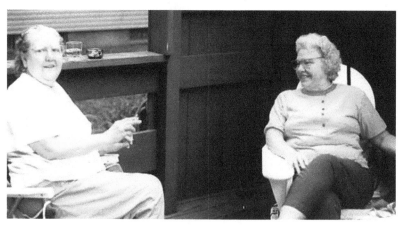

Smoking—Mom on the right and my Aunt
Betty enjoying a smoke together.

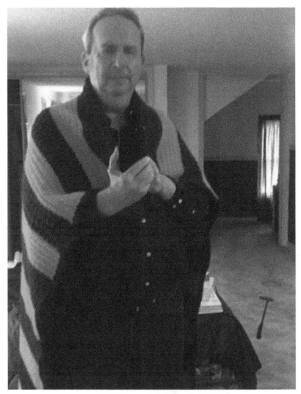

Shawl—Months later I broke out the Prayer Shawl for a picture
for this book. It did the job! I'm strong enough now to
think about golf. I'm in my upstairs putting practice area.

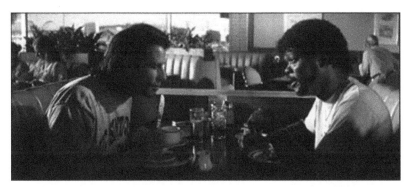

Pulp Fiction—Not from a family album. In 'Pulp Fiction' Jules'
attitude about letting God guide him after saving his life was
odd to his criminal buddy Vincent, but one I could relate to.

Job

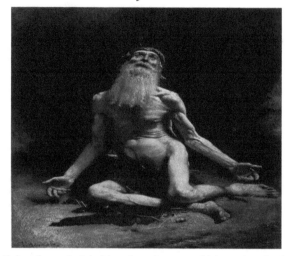

Job acknowledged his fate, but would keep his faith

St Blaise

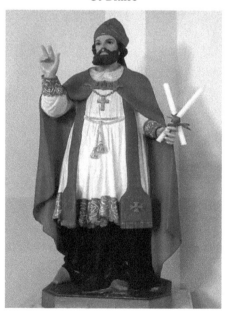

St. Blaise was a bishop and martyr, and perhaps at one time
a physician. The miracle of St Blaise and the blessing of the
throats have propelled the faith since the 8th century.

St Peregrine

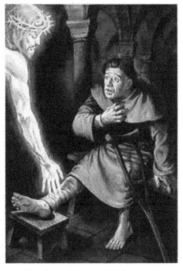

St Peregrine had a vision of Christ coming down from the cross to heal him of his cancer, the night before his leg was to be amputated. That morning the surgeons found no trace of sickness.

St Joseph

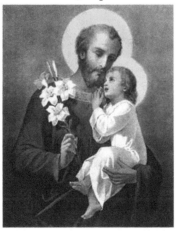

Joseph is a good role model in accepting the will of God that we can all emulate. Pope Francis admires him for his silence and strength.

15. Last Day of Chemo!

March 5, 2018

After last week, I was worried treatments were going to be delayed further. But Doc said blood counts had returned to normal, the chest X-ray Friday showed no more lung build up. *Thanks, Auntie Biotics*, and that we could continue with the last treatment. We went over hydration strategy and new nausea drug regimen to make sure this last treatment goes as smoothly as possible.

It was a long session today. Many people are in the chemo/infusion ward. So many people are in much worse shape than I'm in. A guy next to me was a skeleton with long hair; he mostly just moaned. I said prayers for him and many others passing by (I had a chair really close to the bathroom, which we all had to use a LOT, using our mobile IV units like supportive staffs).

Mortality wise, don't think I've ever been surrounded by so much sickness and death. My late sister, Betty's, chemo treatments in the fall were in her private room. I'm glad she was spared this scene. It *really* made Psalm 23:4 relevant. If I live to be one hundred, I hope I won't ever hear it without thinking back to today.

"Yea, though I walk through the valley of the shadow of death, I will fear no evil: for thou art with me; thy rod and thy staff they comfort me..."

And coming home instead of going back to a hospital room is the *best!*

Humming this little snippet since being back!
Home, home again.

Pink Floyd, Time

Six more days of radiation before I get to ring the bell :-).

Comments:

Patrick O'D.

Hang in there Eddie, you continue to be in our prayers

Pattie S.

Here with you, Eddie! Thought you'd enjoy knowing that I was at OLA fish fry this past Friday. When people learned I was Betty's cousin, they came over to tell funny stories. I learned a hilarious one about a Red star stamp that she used for people who were a pain in the rear (she was the cashier and after payment forwarded the orders). They thought she was giving them a red star because they were special, but in reality she was forewarning the kitchen staff!

Extended version:

This video was very short, just a portion of a longer tune, "Time." It showed a shot of the band closing in gradually on David Gilmour, with the lyrics displayed like a karaoke screen. "Home, home again / I like to be here when I can." After an extended stay in the hospital, I was grateful for being home again.

I had some seriously good mojo going into my last chemo treatment. Being in the hospital and receiving extra meds helped with my attitude to literally "hang out" with my chemo drugs on the mobile stand next to me, in an extremely busy infusion center filled with desperate patients and angel nurses doing their best to make people comfortable.

It would not be my last visit there by any means. After recognizing the importance of hydration to prevent constipation and the resultant complications, I insisted on using the infusion center to pump saline solution into me five times a week. I was coming to the hospital five days a week anyway for radiation treatments, so I figured to use all the resources I could to get well. It was a fast way to get half my hydration daily requirements, and then depending on my energy level, I would do as much as possible at home. My goal was 150 percent of the required hydration.

> *"but whoever drinks of the water that I will give him shall never thirst; but the water that I will give him will become in him a well of water springing up to eternal life"* (John 4:14).

Sometimes you have to be aggressive with your own treatment plan and not go with the status quo. I wanted the poison from the chemo flushed out of my system as quickly as possible as did they. And since I was increasing antibiotics from the previous week's complication, I knew constipation could reoccur from those, even though antibiotics were part of the cocktail mix of chemotherapy I was getting. The team was very cooperative and gave me no resistance to the increase. Some of the staff actually said they liked it when patients take responsibility for knowing their conditions and make sound suggestions to get themselves well.

In the previous six months, I had read a book on conditioning by quarterback, Tom Brady, who is the oldest, most successful quarterback in the NFL today. He had a whole chapter on hydration and attributes his ability to quickly bounce back from brutal collisions week after week during the season to proper hydration. In *Saving Private Ryan*, Tom Hank's character, Captain Miller, was constantly swigging out of his canteen. Basic army training teaches that dehydration is a soldier's worst enemy. A Led Zeppelin tune entitled "No Quarter" talks about using the path where no one goes. Despite the dreary atmosphere of the infusion center, where this took place, I was determined not to fall victim to dehydration. I would give no quarter

70

to cancer, and that included taking command from the hospital (or it could be an insurance company) for a change in standard treatment.

Psalm 23:4 was in this day's daily liturgy, perfect for what I was going through. The mobile hydration stand was, indeed, a staff that supported myself and others in walking around the infusion center. It was also the staff that supported the many bags of chemicals that would help make us well, God willing.

16. Beginning of the End of Treatments

March 11, 2018

This week, I have my last two radiation treatments. The radiation will be resonating in my throat region for a while—everyone is different—still burning out the cancer. But at least, no more direct hits, and I will let you know how it goes. Chemo is done, but this next week is the last danger period from that when my immunity is at its nadir (bottom). Hope everyone has good weather and does some corned beef for me on St. Pats! Next year, we'll party big time!

An Irish parish down the street from me, St. Mel's, introduced me to this prayer to St. Michael. The image on the card is much like the last few battle scenes with Gandalf and a fiery monster in this (YouTube) version of "The Battle of Evermore" by Led Zeppelin. Both call on a higher power to get us through a hard battle. I watched *The Lord of the Rings trilogy* with my sister, Betty, when they first came out. They were some of her favorite films and watched again at the beginning of treatments with her gone only a month. Her memory helps pull me through too.

> *St. Michael the Archangel, defend us in battle. Be our defense against the wickedness and snares of the devil. May God rebuke him, we humbly pray, and do you, O prince of the heavenly host, by the power*

of God, thrust into hell Satan and all the evil spirits
who prowl about the world seeking the ruin of souls.
Amen.

Comments:

Uncle Bob

Loved the music. I almost got my walker and started dancing! Eddie, you are my inspiration. Prayers and love continue hourly! Go Cavs!

Annie A.

Sweet prayer! Seeing light at the end of the tunnel big bro! You are awesome! See you soon! Xoxoxo

Extended version:

Police and firemen have the toughest jobs in the world. Of course, I'm a bit biased because my dad was a cop. He and many of his comrades were required to live in the city of Cleveland, and so our neighborhood parish and many of the others nearby adopted the prayer above into their church services, whereby all their family and neighbors could pray for the safety of our safety forces.

Only God knows why some people get cancer and some don't. When you have it though, you're battling against something you can't see except in X-rays. Something pretty much invisible, like an evil spirit. The importance of imagery can't be understated. You have to focus on your daily regimen, discipline yourself to a healthy lifestyle, skip going out for major celebrations temporarily.

Luckily during this time, I could still pick teams for the NCAA brackets. Usually I was the "Commish" at work, coordinating our library's bracket competition using CBS Sports free app. This year, I delegated it. This was the first time in my adult life that I was able to watch the whole championship, and they provided a great distraction. But thanks to fatigue, it was a struggle staying awake for all the games!

Distracting yourself from the effects of treatment sometimes takes effort. Sometimes God blesses you and delivers a distraction that takes no effort to take advantage of, some kind of sight, sound, or companionship! Both distraction and positive action should be part of any personal treatment plan. My dad always says he thinks doctors overmedicate. I think that's true to a degree. You do need some drugs, but the patient has to come up with ways of their own to at least *feel* well in their own minds.

Maybe you can't strike out at a monster with a sword like Gandalf did, but you can take steps to prevent that Mean Ol' Cancer and its ally, depression, from hurting your chances of getting well. You can strike back by surrounding yourself with inspiring quotes, music, and video. Today's song, "The Battle of Evermore," combined all three!

The person producing this YouTube music video did a fantastic job of editing scenes from *The Lord of the Ring* movies, synchronizing them with phrases of the song; Gandalf's struggle with the monster in the last third captured the essence of my own fight.

> "At last, the sun is shining, the clouds of blue roll by, / With flames from the dragon of darkness, / The sunlight blinds his eyes."
> Led Zeppelin, The Battle of Evermore

Be creative. You and your caregivers—your allies in this battle—can figure out ways to keep your health and spirits up. One person I know, Annie, who lost her hair due to chemo, had a cool, intricate henna tattoo replace her hair—much better than a scarf in warm weather. It looked good and gave a statement about not being down due to baldness. She might not have a flaming sword like Gandalf did, but this action was her weapon.

Friends who knew I was bumming about my missing St. Patrick's Day sent me St. Patrick's Day cards. Phil and Nancy in Colorado sent me a Chieftains music CDs, Kerryman jokes (offensive if you're from Kerry, funny to all other Irish folks; interchangeable with any ethnic group, totally not PC) and a great book, *How the Irish Saved*

Civilization by Thomas Cahill. Isolated monks on the Island copied by hand, volumes of ancient Greek and Roman texts. Each card and gift received by me were an arrow in my quiver against cancer, like the arrows the character Daryl uses in "The Walking Dead."

> "*You went down so that you can come up, you cried so that you can rejoice, you mourned so that you can dance, you did without so that you can overcome, you want to tell every devil in hell. Somebody holler the fight is on*" (T.D. Jakes).

Holy cards of St. Michael always show him with a sword. Create your own swords! Make distraction and positive action part of your personal treatment plan.

17. Here's to a Bright Future!

March 14, 2018

I'm all done now with the radiation treatments and rang the bell yesterday as I was leaving. My brother, Tom, who has driven me a ton of times to treatments requested this tune to celebrate! "The Future's So Bright" by Timbuk 3.

I will still be going in daily for at least two more weeks for hydration treatments but will never have to wear the head mask again! Hopefully by then, the effects of the radiation will have worn out enough that I can swallow liquids. Right now, I do one thousand milliliter of saline in hydration and another one thousand at home through the PEG tube when I can. It's about sixty-seven liquid ounces. Thanks to all for your continuing support. My energy level is still low, but I mean to get individually back to each and every one of you soon!

> "I'm heavenly blessed and worldly wise / I'm a peeping-tom techy with X-ray eyes / Things are going great, and they're only getting better / I'm doing all right, getting good grades / The future's so bright, I gotta wear shades"
>
> Timbuk 3, The Future's So Bright.

Comments:

Patricia H.

GOD IS GOOD!! Hang in there and receive all the Blessings coming your way. You have a great Brother supporting you. Pat

Kathy J.

Perfect song! So, so proud of the way you've dealt with this challenge! Let the healing begin! xxxooo

Extended version:

This was a trippy video from the MTV days; cartoon GIFs and musicians faking playing in the desert next to a *Breaking Bad*-like mobile home, with a donkey here and there for laughs. In a silly, happy mood after ringing the bell, at the time I'm sure this was a great New Year's Eve party song. It totally fits! Leave it to my cool brother to come up with it!

> "*Always laugh when you can. It is cheap medicine*"
> (Lord Byron).

Getting through with radiation treatments didn't mean being through with the hospital. As I wrote—thanks to changing my hydration schedule—I would still be coming back daily. I can't imagine how much slower the recovery process would've been if I hadn't started doing extra hydration.

As the weeks progressed, I'd start sending out snail mail thank-you cards from home for all the folks supporting me through CaringBridge, snail mail, and dropping by and through phone calls. My chances of infection started dropping a few weeks after chemo (or so I thought), so a few more folks did drop by, and I started going out myself to stores for cards, etc.

The radiation center must be a really tough place to work. Most patients I saw tried to be cheerful, but you could see, in some eyes and in the eyes of their caregivers, desperation. Some simply had a resigned look on their faces, probably rightfully so because they had accepted the inevitable and were just going through the motions of treatment to prolong life for someone else's sake, not theirs.

The radiation staff, like the infusion center staff, are like angels. At least they were at my hospital, and I have to believe they're everywhere else. Mine were always looking out for my comfort with heated blankets while I was on the table (more like a bed), where I laid under the radiation machine, always looking forward to what tunes I would bring in. They all gathered when I rang the bell, and in hindsight, I wish we would've gotten a picture with everyone. When I rang the bell, I realized that it wasn't just me celebrating. It was good for their morale as well.

Midway through the treatments, a horrible incident dealing with the loss of thousands of frozen embryos had occurred at one of their other hospitals in an unrelated department. But it was on the news every night for weeks, and I'm sure they were all affected. It's tough enough, I'm sure, administering treatments that over time take away people's hair, appetite, mobility, and God knows what else, and then have the media stigma to deal with. I did my best to help keep them in good spirits as they did me. Like a team that's struggling at halftime, they needed encouragement. I think any radiation team needs that, due to the nature of their work, not just due to tragedy, and that love goes around. They provide it to the patients; the patients return it to them is how the Big Guy I think would like to see it go. The world is always a better place when love is reciprocal. I can't help believing that buoying up your medical team causes a reciprocity that creates a positive synergy which contributes to the curative process.

> "And in the end, the love you take, is equal to the love you make"
> The Beatles, Paul McCartney, The End.

18. Family Thoughts

March 19, 2018

I had a lot of family in town doing stuff this weekend, most of which I missed due to the nasty side effects still going on from treatment. Still good hearing from everyone and seeing how we support each other.

Today's the feast day of St. Joseph, husband of Mary. The prayer after communion service echoes my thoughts for all the Rossmans, Andrakos, Pinardos, and Skrahs, who make up my great clan!

> *"Defend with unfailing protection, O Lord we pray, the family you have nourished with food from this alter, as they rejoice at the Solemnity of St. Joseph, and graciously keep safe your gifts among them. Through Christ our Lord. Amen."*

When I was on the road for twelve years, cruising all over the country, this song would always remind me of and help me appreciate my family and home.

> The voices talking somewhere in the house, late spring / And you're drifting off to sleep with your teeth in your mouth / You are here with me / You are here with me / You have been here and you are everything.
>
> R.E.M., You Are The Everything

Comments:

Virginia S.

The sun is shining today—I hope you are near a window. Warmth from the sun always gives us extra strength to journey on and I hope you will feel that way all day today!!!!

Sending prayers and love your way,
Virginia

Fern B.

Family and friends are everything. Sending good thoughts.

Extended version:

I think it's natural that when you have cancer or any life-threatening disease that you look back into the past to a better time before when you had the disease, before when you could do the things healthy people take for granted. There were many nights as a child where I would drift off to sleep listening to my mom talking on the phone in the kitchen to her sister, my Aunt Betty Pinardo (who my sister was named after), while my dad worked a late-night police shift. It was a comforting memory for me as an adult, a time when I was healthy (with your teeth in your mouth) and protected. Now I know Mom's calls to her sister weren't just chatter but their way of giving each other support while Dad was out facing down bad guys and my Uncle Nick worked late hours at his popular Italian nightclub. Sibling support, I think, is one of the strongest forces in the world!

Now's the time where families put things aside and try to help each other out. Frankly, as a single guy, I had done a lot of travelling in my youth, and the "preoccupation" of family was never that important to me as the fun of experiencing life was. My wanderlust was pretty powerful, but I was pleasantly surprised that when sickness came, how many of my family popped up to wish me well. We never had any feuds, just distance and different priorities. It is a shame that it takes cancer to overcome that.

Joseph is the model of a man accepting God's will that we can all emulate. I'm sure he was shocked by the news that his virgin fiancée was expecting. Even more stunned when an angel told him that she'd conceived—thanks to the Holy Spirit—and her child should be named Jesus. But he accepted the word of God and would do his best protecting his family by escaping Herod and going to Egypt. Then raising Jesus as his own and teaching him the carpentry trade.

> *"I have great love for Saint Joseph, because he is a man of silence and strength. On my table I have an image of Saint Joseph sleeping. Even when he is asleep, he is taking care of the Church! Yes! We know that he can do that. So when I have a problem, a difficulty, I write a little note and I put it underneath Saint Joseph, so that he can dream about it! In other words I tell him: pray for this problem!"* (Pope Francis).

Joseph stayed in the here and now, accepting the will of God and proceeding as best he could with his family. We—struck by cancer—need to do the same thing. We have a great role model in St. Joseph, to accept what life has dealt us and do the best we can for our clan.

19. Post Radiation Syndrome

April 4, 2018

Was I wrong? Radiation treatment ended three weeks ago, and I knew effects would still be reverberating but didn't anticipate how slow the process would be. Last few weeks filled w/ a lot of coughing and fatigue. I have definitely seen *Better Days*.

I 'm gradually getting better though, actually was able to start sipping Powerade and not feeling like I was swallowing razor blades this week.

Doing a lot of dozing with my prayer shawl my sister, Ann, brought up for me from Florida. A great organization, the St. Thomas Stitchers Prayer Shawl Ministry, has a circle that creates nice warm shawls for the sick and includes with them a shawl prayer:

> *I call nine blessings from above. In the name of God, the Creator, the Giver of Life, the Holder of time. In the name of Jesus, the Savior, the Healer and the Lifter of Pain, in the name of the Spirit, the Comforter, the Counselor, the Sustainer of Life. I wear a mantle of caring. I wear a mantle of protection. I wear a mantle of wholeness. I wear a mantle of strength. I wear a mantle of healing. I wear a mantle of patience. I wear a mantle to enfold me. I wear a mantle to encircle me. I wear a mantle to empower me.*

At Shaker Library, the lady who championed in starting our knitting circles, Fern Braverman, lost her husband from a long illness just before the holidays. I'm sending her prayers to ease her sorrow.

> "I'm faded, flat busted / Been jaded, I been dusted / I know that I've seen better days"
> Citizen King, Better Days

Comments:

Wendy S.

Hoping with each new day you are feeling better, stronger and more comfortable. Sending healing thoughts and wishes your way.

Sandy P.

Ed, we are glad that you see signs that you are healing. What a gift from Annie! It's bringing you comfort. One day at a time, Cousin! Constant prayers, Nick and Sandy

Extended version:

In my front room, where I spent most of my time during the day, I had hung over the couch a Cleveland Browns blanket that I would take to the stadium with me and dates to help keep them warm in our seats. During the winter of 2018, the Browns had just come out of a 0–16 season. Ugh. Getting this new shawl was a great replacement! It was as good as the Browns getting our new quarterback in the draft, Baker—Baker "Touchdown Maker" Mayfield.

Being sick as I was, I was also pretty self-conscious. I needed a portable spittoon. I used a large metallic car coffee mug to walk everywhere with because I was constantly coughing up phlegm. Even though it was a positive sign of healing, my "sunburned" throat was basically oozing out healing lubricant; it was pretty messy. So I found myself, before getting the shawl, sitting on my couch, trying to read, trying to watch TV, but constantly dozing. Fatigue was produced by the healing process, I guess. Terribly interrupted sleep and lack of proper nutrition kept me sidelined for days, or should I say "daze."

The shawls' arrival could not have come at a better time! I love each line of the prayer. God being the Holder of time. I've never thought of Him that way before, making things like recovery go fast or slow, "thy kingdom come, thy will be done," or the unexpected gift of the shawl coming just as I needed it! Jesus being the Lifter of pain. I think this stage of recovery was especially hard because normal expectations would be that things would immediately get better, part of our instant gratification culture, I guess. The Holy Spirit being the Comforter, Counselor, and Sustainer, giving me the strength to weather this storm.

Mantle can be defined two ways: as an article of clothing and as a role of responsibility. The six characteristics symbolized virtues that can be asked for and acted on. Caring, protection, wholeness, strength, healing, and patience were all things I could try to do to lift myself out of the self-imposed bubble of isolation I was in. The shawl I kept on like a talisman, something that would cover me physically and empower me spiritually. Giving me the strength to start getting back to each and every post that came into CaringBridge, sending positive vibes to someone going through her own tragedy, replacing fluids through my own body and not through a bag or a tube, and waiting…the hardest part, patiently for God's time, Jesus's mercy, and the Holy Spirit's strength to get me through this period and on to "better days."

20. I Heart Jell-O

April 10, 2018

Just finished my first solid food in over two months! Irish Jell-O, lemon-lime, of course! Felt okay, throat's still scratchy, but after sipping Powerade all week, I figured it was time for an upgrade! Would not be here this quickly if it wasn't for all the great prayers and vibes you were all sending me. Thanks to you and the grace of God, I'm feeling like Chicago sings, "I'm feelin' stronger every day!"

> "Feelin stronger every day [You know I'm alright now] / Feeling stronger every day."
> Chicago, Feelin' Stronger Every Day

Comments:

Tom R.

Way to go Bro—next few months we can do jello shots!

Pattie S.

Green jello is the best!!!

Simone N.

Hello Ed. This is Margaret F. I am thinking and praying for you! Stay strong and may God continue to keep you in his hands. Best regards!!!

Virginia S.

I was so happy to hear that you were eating Jell-O!!!! In honor of Poetry Month, I wanted to send you this poem, "Squishy Touch,", by Shel Silverstein.

Everything King Midas touched turned to gold, the lucky fellow.
Every single thing I touch turns to raspberry (lime) Jell-O.
Today I touched the kitchen wall (squish).
I went and punched my brother, Paul, (splish).
I tried to fix my bike last week (sploosh).
I kissed my mother on the cheek (gloosh).
I tried to read the Evening News (smush).
I sat down in the easy chair (splush).
I tried to comb my wavy hair (slush).
I took a dive into the sea (glush).
Would you like to shake hands with me (sklush)?

Just so you know, Ed, I will shake hands with you anytime!!!!!
Extra prayers are coming your way! (We do miss you around here!)

Extended version:

That was the longest two months ever! All the docs and nurses had been telling me that swallowing is like a muscle exercise, that the body can forget how to do it. When you are healthy, that is hard to imagine, but when your throat has been burned by radiation, it's believable! If you've ever been sunburned on your arms or legs and then had to move them, that's what it's like. Not to mention the discomfort if you're touched! There's no real "Coppertone" or soothing balm you can do either. I was and am still doing mild painkillers like naproxen or Tylenol twenty minutes before trying to use my throat. That helps.

The song, "Stronger Every Day," not just matched my attitude with the lyrics but also with the gradual upbeat tempo of the song. It starts off mellow, then starts building into a high-energy horns, drums, and keyboards frenzy! That's what I was hoping my progress in eating would be like. Starting with Jell-O, then eventually bring on the all-you-can-eat Chinese buffet!

In the aforementioned book, *Burn the Fat, Feed the Muscle* by Tom Venuto, he describes his recommended method of building muscle with weights. Setting an easy baseline, doing that for a week, then progressively adding weights for resistance each week thereafter, being patient but steady in your routine. That way, you gradually get stronger without injuring your body. I tried to follow the same approach to eating. First, a week of sipping Powerade to get used to swallowing again, as well as getting some needed hydration, electrolytes, and vitamins besides my crushed pills and the food tube's liquid nutrition. I'd progress on to Jell-O, then applesauce, then yogurt (much tougher, both in consistency and taste, could not find any with good flavor to my injured taste buds), then KFC mashed potatoes and gravy (tougher consistency, but I loved what I could taste, plus it smelled delicious), and on and on.

> *"If you always put limit on everything you do, physical or anything else. It will spread into your work and into your life. There are no limits. There are only plateaus, and you must not stay there, you must go beyond them"* (Bruce Lee).

In my efforts, I had plenty of cheerleaders. It took a few days, but now I got back to everyone individually who posted a comment to CaringBridge. I received wit and wisdom from friends and family all over the world and felt truly blessed. I knew it would take time, and I was entering into a long season of recovery.

> *"For everything there is a season, and a time for every matter under heaven"* (Ecclesiastes 3:1).

21. Done with Hydration!

April 14, 2018

Another positive step. Met with my oncologist, Thursday, and we decided it was time to quit the hospital hydration and just focus on getting enough liquid through regular food and the PEG-tube cans and gradually weening off those as well. My condition has improved enough that my problems are mostly in the top part of throat and mouth, still building up liquid whenever I exercise the vocal cords. So no longer daily visits to Southwest General Hospital, which I've been doing pretty much since chemo and radiation started last January 22! Ugh.

My dad keeps saying this healing will be a slow process, like watching paint dry. Case in point, Kathy and I celebrated stopping hydration with wonton soup from Dragon Towers at Kamm's Corners. Soup tasted great, but the wontons were a bit like wet cardboard (not the cook's fault, my throat's!). But they didn't hurt going down, so I'm just going to have to keep working those taste buds and staying hydrated until I can taste things normally. Today's daily scripture reading had this quote from St. Francis de Sales that seems appropriate: "*We shall steer safely through every storm, as long as our heart is right, our intention fervent, our courage steadfast, and our trust fixed in God.*"

So now it's a matter of patience, trying foods that I may not like, but that'll help get me well. Like peaches! Those have lots of liquid and should make me stronger, like in this video by the Presidents of the United States of America's "Peaches."

"I'm movin' to the country, / I'm gonna eat me a lot of peaches."

Comments:

Billy C.

Ed—Hope you are getting better every day. Peaches…oddly enough I have heard that song 2 or 3 times in the last week or so…must be a good omen!! I am keeping you in my prayers daily. Take care, Cap

Uncle Bob

Good job Eddie. First the storm then the calm and the peace and the joy and the total healing. Oops, almost forgot the juicy burger combined with the Great Lakes Dortmunder.

Extended version:

This video matched the vibe that was happening to me at this point, regarding eating. It shows the three-man group at first just playing their song in a grove of peach trees, and then all of a sudden they are fighting ninjas, who crept up on them. Good campy special effects, doing some *Matrix*-like leaps and punches but making it look like a fight on the old *Batman* series. They end up beating up the ninjas!

Their struggle was a little like what I was going through, battling the disconnect between how something would smell and how it would actually taste! There was always a little disappointment to go through, even with sweet-smelling juicy peaches because I couldn't really taste them yet. But I knew they were good for me, as were a zillion other broths and foods, so the challenge was to keep trying different things.

As the quote from St. Francis in my CaringBridge comment implies, at this late stage of the game a lot was on me. The medical team has done its thing; now I had to do mine. This was just another storm. To make progress through it I had to be proactive and try different nutrition tactics. I went through grapes, apples, precut cantaloupe and watermelon because I didn't want to invest too much energy in food prep. I tried my favorite canned soup, one of my favorite bar's, Kelley's, homemade beef stroganoff and chicken alfredo that my buddy, CJ's girlfriend, Val, prepared for me with extra sauce. Still no alcohol but trying to drink down various flavors of any drink ending in "ade." Powerade, Gatorade, lemonade, and a few other vitamin beverages. Frequently they tasted like crap or nothing at all. But I could see myself gaining strength, and when something tasted okay, I made sure to get more.

Sometimes when possible if it wasn't right, I gave it away. I gave away a lot more than I kept in the beginning, believe me. But as Og Mandino wrote: "The sailor learns by riding out the wrath of each storm." Eventually I changed my attitude, and unless it was something that burned my throat, like some tomatoes and grapes did in the beginning, I finished things anyway just to get the hydration and nutrients they provided.

> "Nothing worth having comes without some kind of fight/Got to kick at the darkness till it bleeds daylight"
> Bruce Cockburn, Lovers In A Dangerous Time

You have to have a stout heart to keep trying, keeping your eye on the prize of the intention of getting well. Being brave before trying a succulent-smelling juicy rib, knowing there's a good chance it won't taste anything like it smells. Yes, it might totally disappoint you, and if you're weak, it could spin you off into depression, thinking you'll never enjoy food again. It's an exaggerated fear. To overcome it, you have to keep trying and trust in the Lord that over time, you will enjoy his creations again.

22. This Week

April 22, 2018

I've been saying "this week" a lot lately. It's a good coping mechanism as my throat area keeps going through changes and every week, every day actually, something changes. This week, I can talk longer at one time without sipping fluid than I could last week. This week, I can eat more foods than last week. I can't eat grapes, yet something about the juice really irritates my throat…this week. It hurts a bit doing basic chores, thanks to the PEG-tube in my chest… this week. My favorite Progresso soup I leave half-eaten, but I can do a whole can of broth…this week. As time moves on, I know I'll get better and will get back to normal activities and eating, although not too much… I'm at 194 now and would like to stay down there!

This week, I plan to try a little cooking of favorite things like omelet and lemon-basted tilapia. Doc says lemon helps stimulate salivary glands damaged by the radiation and now causing the dry mouth symptoms and taste bud issues. I also read on a cancer blog how zinc helps, so w/ his approval, I'm high dosing on that. And with every taste barrier I break, I sing to myself "Time has come today" by The Chambers Brothers.

The link above goes to a live version, the longest one I could find almost fifteen minutes of psychedelic music. Just the same amount of time it took for me to swap dressings and clean up my PEG tube, a chore I really don't like, looking at the hole in my chest. Playing it helped me through the first dozen times or so, but now I'm finishing much faster than the song. Progress!

Today's mass had this Psalm 116 reading that will be a question I ponder for a while: "*How shall I make a return to the Lord for all the good he has done for me?*"

> Now the time has come, there are things to realize, time has come today.
> The Chambers Brothers, Time Has Come Today—(Live extended version)

Comments:

John H.

I always hated changing my own dressing, I feel your pain on that one. Glad to see progress however small. I remember celebrating being able to tie my own shoes again. Celebrate each step forward.

"How shall I make a return to the Lord for all the good he has done for me?"

Just talk to Him on a daily basis, thank Him for what He has given you & share your hopes and dreams with Him. He is listening…He is your best friend.

Extended version:

This entry's theme was all about time management. After months of treatment and being on the mend, the concept of time as a tool really came into focus for me, both physically and more importantly mentally. The mantra, "this week," is something I still use to give myself and others around me hope that things will be getting better. Maybe derivative of the classic "this too will pass," it was my way of telling myself and others what was happening to me in the "now" and leaving a safety valve for improvement. As I became better and came into contact with more people asking about my condition, I felt I could openly tell them what was going good or bad but include "this week" as a sign of optimism.

The lyric, "time has come today," was something I'd previously sing whenever I made a great (read lucky) golf shot in previous seasons. The song has always been a favorite, and I had it on some mixtapes I made when I used music in the gym or outside to help me run or bike faster.

I never looked forward to changing the dressing around the PEG tube, even though I knew it was important to stop infection. It was awkward, messy, not painful, but sufficiently weird when I accidently would lose hold of the tube, and it would tug in my insides thanks to gravity pulling it down. So I started playing various long tunes to make it a better experience, much like playing tunes helped during radiation. I settled on this one because it took roughly fourteen minutes to take the tape off the gauze, take that off and dispose of it, clean any dried ooze, clean around the insertion point just below the solar plexus, spread antibiotic cream on and around the wound, replace fresh gauze and re-tape. When I started this process while singing and head bopping to "Time Has Come Today," it actually became fun. Something I would do around the same time every day and not blow off.

"Do what you should do, when you should do it, whether you feel like it or not" (Thomas Huxley).

Time management included pondering life after this was over. The day's line from Psalm 116:12, *"How shall I make a return to the Lord for all the good he has done for me?"* had me think of the future. Like the namesake of *Saving Private Ryan*, this line boils down to wondering how I will earn being saved, dodging the bullet, and being rescued. This whole cancer experience brings this question into a realm beyond the theoretical theological question. It's something I ask and try to answer every day now.

I've turned the question into a quest. The destination is payback to the Lord for saving me when many others have died. The route on my quest will be up to me. And with the time I have left, I plan on making it a great adventure!

23. Minor Setback

April 26, 2018

Imagine my surprise yesterday when I tried feeding myself through the tube, and it didn't work! Worked on it for thirty minutes. Luckily, I was able to contact the doc's office who put it in. They saw me right away and determined that the stomach end of the tube got dislodged and was in the abdominal wall. Not a good thing.

They scheduled me for surgery asap, pulled it out, and replaced it. Was home in time for the Cav's victory but dozed a few times thanks to lingering anesthesia effects. Saw the end though, an amazing athletic feat by LeBron. Game saving block then a tie breaking three-pointer from midcourt to win the game! Slept for twelve hours afterward. I'm happy that I'd done all my major house and estate chores I needed to do earlier this week. Can't think about driving today, still pretty sore, but energy level is much better.

Aggravated though, had been making a lot of progress. Feeling a little like Cleveland guy, Trent Reznor, in this Nine Inch Nails video, "We're In This Together," caught up in a wave, confused, and angry. But like this note I have in my home office bulletin board states, I know this should make me stronger. I suppose that's why I put it up there for the bad days.

Become a Spiritual Athlete. Occasionally God lets us face trials that strengthen us, much as a successful athlete is conditioned by training. So it may help to think of problems as spiritual conditioning.

"Do not regard lightly the discipline of the Lord, nor lose courage when you are punished by him. For the Lord disciplines him who he loves..." (Hebrews 12:5–6).

Comments:

Eliza R.

Wow Eddie. You're my HERO! Stay strong! Xx Eliza

Uncle Bob

"Therefore I will trust YOU always, though I may seem to be lost I will not fear, for YOU are ever with me, and will never leave me to face my perils alone." Thomas Merton.

Extended version:

I'm grateful that I was able to go three months without a malfunction in the food tube. I was getting better, even driving a little, getting ready to go back to work, not to the operating room again! All my lucky stars must've been aligned correctly because the doctor and surgery team were available to correct the problem. Should've had someone play the lottery for me that day between the successful surgery and Cavaliers basketball game; I was on a roll!

I didn't think of the episode being "punishment" for trying to do too much too soon, although that was the case. I was raking debris out of the yard, grocery shopping, and pushing baskets long distances in Walmart parking lots for exercise, sweeping out the garage...doing things that restored a sense of normalcy and hurt a little bit, but no pain, no gain, right? Wrong. You can't give into being tempted to push yourself physically when you have plastic tubes hanging out of your body, unless the doctors tell you to.

There is room in your life when recovering from cancer for both spiritual and physical conditioning. They say patience is a virtue.

One of several listed by St. Paul in Galatians 5:22–23: "*But the fruit of the Spirit is love, joy, peace, forbearance, kindness, goodness, faithfulness, gentleness, and self-control. Against such things, there is no law.*"

Here he uses the word *forbearance*. A word meaning patient self-control, restraint, and tolerance. Having cancer requires forbearance to get well. Injured athletes know this too, just ask Tiger Woods, who overcame a terrible back condition to win The Master's golf tournament in 2019. Or anyone who has ever had a knee replaced! You will be feeling amazing when getting better and starting to sample life again. But you can't go after it all at once, otherwise, like I did, you end up back in the operating room. Castaneda's *Don Juan* includes forbearance in his four attributes of warriorship, "control, discipline, forbearance, and timing." You have to learn to pace your physical activity so that when it is the right time, it can be fully released.

> "*At the end of the day, scrambling is not just a way to win football games. It is a means of facing life head-on with dedication and persistence, and tenaciously striving to overcome life's inevitable struggles or defeats*" (Bernie Kosar).

Let this be a warning! Don't try to recover too quickly. Allow your support group to help you with chores. You will be back to normal soon enough. When you are faced with a mishap, whether you created it or not, look at it like a challenge from the Lord to turn it into a positive situation. Like the Nine Inch Nails' song says, in a worst-case scenario for the spiritual athlete, you have to hold on.

> "All that we were is gone we have to hold on / when all our hope is gone we have to hold on / all that we were is gone but we can hold on / you and me / we're in this together now / none of them can stop us now / we will make it through somehow."
>
> Nine Inch Nails, We're In This Together

24. Back to Work!

May 1, 2018

I'm on light duty half time (20 hours) this week. Yesterday, my throat was sore afterward, in a good way, from all the talking with my coworkers at the Bertram Woods branch. It was great seeing everyone. Lynne said she heard a lot of squealing and cheering down the hall and knew I must've walked in! It was nice, especially after being "home alone" for so long. First reference question was about starting a nonprofit! A good sign. It was nice being able to go into the stacks and zero in on books that will help them out. To me, that's what librarianship is about. No, I didn't pitch my own book, ha ha.

Today at the Main Library was the same, but I had a chance to work alone in the office more instead of being on the floor, so feeling better—throat wise. Information overload has been going on and chemo brain blocking some name recall, but everyone's taking it in stride. As the Grateful Dead say, "Every silver lining has a touch of grey."

> "Sorry that you feel that way, the only thing there is to say / Every silver lining's got a touch of grey / I will get by / I will get by / I will get by / I will survive."
>
> Grateful Dead, Touch of Grey

In other big news, got the word today, I'll be getting a PET scan next week! That and a couple more diagnostic scopes should give me the word on if I need any more treatments. It will be a challenge not thinking about the outcome, repeating the past few tough months, and instead focusing on work, my sister's estate details, various other important life issues. Need to keep in mind this quote from Proverbs 4:25: *"Let your eyes look straight ahead, and your gaze be focused forward."*

Comments:

Annie A.

Take it Easy (Eagles) Bro! Glad you are getting out and about more and prayers for the upcoming Scans/scopes!!

Jim R.

Great to hear you are back on the job! Thinking of you in the BK. Warm thoughts, Jim

Extended version:

Most music fans know the skeleton is a favorite symbol of the Grateful Dead. This video used some amazing puppets that were look-alike versions of the band members playing this song in concert. Apparently filmed "live in front of an audience," according to the Youtube comments. Very cool video for a very cool song, one of my favorites. It's funny, cynically real, yet strong in faith and optimism. A survivor's song if ever there was one.

As I allude to in my CaringBridge comments, my silver lining and touch of grey was getting back to seeing folks I worked with and basking in their love and attention. I talked a lot and can see why politicians come up with talking points or job hunters use fast "elevator pitches." I went through a lot of throat lozenges those first few days, repeating myself many times on treatment, current condition, and recovery plans. Plus walking around and thanking all those who were part of the CaringBridge platform, my support team.

After a while, I found it best to be brief, factual, and optimistic, not saying even to my bosses that it wasn't confirmed that I wasn't out of the danger zone yet. No use bringing anyone down, I thought. But I was looking to get the PET scan and other diagnostic tests over with soon.

A positron emission tomography (PET) scan is where you're injected with dye, in my case a glucose solution (cancer cells like glucose, if you need a reason to avoid sugar), and then see where it clusters in the body. In my case, it was a head-to-hip scan. They wanted to make sure the cancer hadn't traveled anywhere.

Any cancer patient can identify with this stage of the game. You've been through hell, now is the question "is it over," "have you won," or "are you going into overtime?" Sometimes that's necessary for a victory, but all patients would prefer not reliving the last few months of treatment. One of my favorite horror stories ends with a character going back to the beginning of the tale, crying for "Mercy! Not again!" Doomed, he feared, to an endless loop.

No question that it's human to have that fear despite all the positive reinforcement you and others give to yourself. That's what makes this proverb so perfect, so powerful for recovery:

"Let your eyes look straight ahead, and your gaze be focused forward" (Proverbs 4:25).

25. The Latest Storm

May 6, 2018

Just when I thought I was getting better, an infection spread around the PEG-tube area in my chest that just had a new one put in last week. I've been doing antibiotics, but the bugs must've thought they were vitamins because they grew wider around the tube insertion point. Doc Newton was surprised and ordered a CT scan stat on Friday afternoon to see if its inside me too. No word yet, should find out tomorrow the next steps.

A different doc, Dr. Mendpara, my oncologist, had said he would like me to get the tube out in June due to the possibility of infection, so I guess it's not uncommon. Dr. M was just a month off! I still need it for nutrition. Did discover a new favorite food, pancakes with lots of syrup. Could taste them really well and went down easy!

Just have to grin and bear this infection for now. As Psalm 37.23 says, *"The steps of a good man are ordered by the LORD, and He delighteth in his way."* He's doing it for a reason I guess, maybe that I pace myself in this recovery mode. I do tend to push myself. Almost went to a bar for the first time on Friday to meet Larry and other friends I haven't seen since last year. Probably not a good plan…this week! I will just have to do what the band, Kansas, recommends and "carry on."

Carry on, you will always remember. / Carry on, none can equal the splendor. / Now your life's no longer empty. / Surely heaven waits for you. / Carry on, my wayward son. / There'll be peace when you are done. / Lay your weary head to rest. / Don't you cry (Don't you cry no more). / No more.

Kansas, Carry On My Wayward Son

Comments:

Pattie S.

Great song to inspire!

Cindy M.

Four steps forward, one back. Still making progress!

Extended version:

This is a great song no matter what trials you are going through. This particular version I liked because it's karaoke style, a black background with white lyrics, very easy to read, and every stanza is great, although I like the one above the best. It matches the Psalm reading for that day.

Of course, I was a bit disappointed about the infection but had been warned about it. Remembering my chemo class in January, they'd warned me about the susceptibility to infections cancer patients had. An open wound, like around the PEG tube, was a great target for germs. Apparently my diligence for keeping it clean, or my recent movement from a closed environment like home to an open environment like a public library triggered the infection. Luckily I got right on it and did not choose to be macho and suck it up, waiting for it to be healed on its own. I'd been proactive throughout this whole cancer thing, so I sought treatment, called in sick again from work for a few days, and went into diagnostic mode with the CT-Scan (pronounced cat, as in cat scratch fever, scan).

Actually called a computerized tomography scan, CT scan for short, it's where they put you in a cylinder on your back and move you back and forth, taking X-rays from multiple angles of the area in question. I'd had them in the early days of my treatment. Felt like déjà vu all over again from the beginning, except now I was much more confident that it was searching for a nonlethal invisible infection rather than an invisible, evasive lethal tumor. Thank, goodness, it showed negative, and the doctors prescribed steroidal creams to reduce the infections' effects on my chest and wound.

The infection was probably a good thing, because it caused me to slow down and not do too much, an issue I've written about before. The "First Friday" services would just have to wait, although I did miss seeing the great guys and gals who'd supported me through CaringBridge. I'd buy them a beer next month!

I still made it to mass with my dad and brother, Tom, though; something I hadn't done in a few months due to fear of infection. And after one of these at our traditional post-mass dinners, usually at a nearby Bob Evans or Perkins, I graduated from liquid diet to softer foods. Bacon, I found I could actually taste, although it was tough chewing and swallowing! And although eggs went down okay, they had no taste despite everything I could add to them, peppers, cheese, salsa, nothing registered yet. What I really enjoyed was pancakes. I was at the lowest weight I'd been in decades and still going down, so pancakes coated in butter and syrup became my go-to dinner for another month. Discoveries like this prompted me to start weaning myself from the PEG tube. And after the infection, I could see its days being numbered!

Again, the mantra, "this week," came into play when running into roadblocks like the infection, as well as minor victories like enjoying pancakes and bacon. The Psalm reading I used in CaringBridge was a good one for this stormy period, and in reflection now, I could've added the next line: "*The steps of a good man are ordered by the LORD: and He delighteth in his way. Though he fall, he shall not be utterly cast down: for the LORD upholdeth him with his hand*" (Psalm 32:23–24).

Even though I applied as much of the chemo class lessons as I could and thought I was pacing myself, I still got hit with an infection. Yes, it itched, looked large and purple and scared everyone seeing it. But it would be treatable. It didn't go internal, infecting my stomach and other organs.

There's a current hit movie on cable now called *Bird Box*, where people have to wear a blindfold to avoid seeing some unknown alien demons that cause people to kill themselves. Cancer treatments are like this. Unless you're a medical person, you're blinded by science, taking the steps the doctors tell you to take. You can, however, trust in the Lord that he has planned for each step you need, whispering in your ear the direction physically and spiritually you should follow. Even if you have to "go long." And if you do this, you may trip up and skin your knees, maybe even break a leg. But in the end, He'll guide you through each storm you face.

26. Celebrate!

May 13, 2018

Went to Dr. Shah, the doc who first diagnosed and removed the malignant tumor from my neck, who reviewed the PET scan test and said all was back to normal! I have one more doc to see next week and many more follow-ups over the months and years ahead as any cancer patient does, but it looks like I'm out of the proverbial cancer woods!!!!

As Rare Earth sings, "I just want to celebrate."

> Well, I can't be bothered with sorrow / And I can't be bothered with hate, no, no / I'm using up the time but feeling fine, every day / That's why I'm telling you I just want to celebrate / Oh, yeah / I just want to celebrate another day / Oh, I just want to celebrate another day of livin' / I just want to celebrate another day of life.

"May the God of hope fill you with all joy and peace in believing" (Romans 15:13).

Comments:

Mary O.

Celebrate, celebrate, dance to the music!
Thank God.

Uncle Bob

So thank you God, for listening to my troubles and anxiety. Have a good day God, I love You, too. And I will call again tomorrow. All my trust is in You!

Cindy M.

Hallelujah!

George B.

Amen!!!

Extended version:

This great song matched my spirit exactly and no doubt many others. The video is simply the album cover, where this song appeared, "One Earth," but the YouTube comments are priceless. The first I saw was from another cancer survivor! Others ranged from soldiers in Afghanistan to people celebrating their birthdays, rejoicing in this high energy song from the seventies!

After Dr. Shah examined the PET scan results, he did one more procedure to make sure, a diagnostic laryngoscopy. He used a fiber-optic camera through my nose and into the throat. Yes, he numbed the area first and had me blow out any buggers I could then went in. It took about five minutes but felt a lot longer, and felt as good as a nose squeeze by Moe in the Three Stooges. He apologized for any discomfort, but I told him and his nurse what has become one of my favorite lines in this whole ordeal: "No pain, no gain." That had them both chuckle.

I don't think they're used to supportive comments from their patients. The people I saw in their waiting room were usually sourpusses, and I heard at times over the months people badgering staff over appointments or bills or flat-out panicked screams from being probed, prodded, and picked at to remove wax from plugged ears or whatever procedures they were into an ear, nose, and throat office for. The least I could do was not make my "team" there feel bad about doing their jobs and helping me become well.

My brother, Tom, went with me, and after, we walked next door to an Irish bar, PJ McIntyres, where my friend Doug poured my first beer, a Guinness Stout and I tried some Shepherd's Pie. A fine way to celebrate! Shepard's Pie is a ground beef and vegetable casserole-type dish topped off by mashed potatoes. Perfect for someone in my still raw condition to eat. But doctor's orders! Had to start building up those swallowing muscles. I finished the beer but not the food. It became one of what would become many take-home boxes for me over the next few months as I experimented with different foods.

My weight had sunk to 193, probably the lowest in over twenty years!

My CaringBridge comment was pretty short, and on doing research for this book, which I hadn't thought about doing at the time, I found that I cut it in half. The full quotation is:

"May the God of hope fill you with all joy and peace in believing, so that by the power of the Holy Spirit you may abound in hope" (Romans 15:13).

As I discovered through this experience, the power of the Holy Spirit helped a lot, especially overcoming the feelings of survival guilt. I'd seen a lot of death and discomfort due to cancer over the last few months, including my own dear sister, and fellow patients in the radiation waiting room, chemo and infusion center. Even in this day's packed ear, nose, and throat waiting room, there were a lot of people with crabby attitudes. I could survive this ordeal without losing a good attitude, giving up a seat when needed, trying to be friendly and being a good role model for both the adults and children there.

Time on earth is like one big waiting room, I realized. A lot of trials and tribulation, but with the power of the Holy Spirit, you can keep your peace, be generous to others, and not live your precious life whining and being a victim. Hope neutralizes that negativity and helps me celebrate like the song says, "another day of livin'."

27. Unplugged! Final Entry

May 23, 2018

I had my PEG tube removed yesterday. No painkiller, the sadist. It reminded me of removing a bike tube from a tight bike rim, getting most of it except the nozzle, where you put the air in, pulling it and then *thwack!* It comes out. It sounded and felt like that, a hard slap from inside my stomach. But I'm glad it's out.

It was just about the last part of the cancer treatment to deal with. I still have a port in my upper chest that'll stay with me a few years and needs a flush every six weeks, but that's nothing—pain wise.

This'll be the final entry. Thanks again for all your encouraging comments over the last few months. I have been a little slack on responding, but I love you all and know your good thoughts and prayers helped me survive this.

The whole experience has made me see life differently, and I'm looking forward to making the most of it. But as a sign I suppose...today's Mass's first Bible reading was about not boasting about tomorrow.

> *Come now, you who say, "Today or tomorrow we will go to this or that city, spend a year there, carry on business, and make a profit." You do not even know what will happen tomorrow! What is your life? You are a mist that appears for a little while and then vanishes. Instead, you ought to say, "If the Lord is willing, we will live and do this or that. (James 4:13–14)*

And if the Lord is willing, He'll give me the time and energy to continue doing what another Boss sings about, being "Born to Run." Go Cavs! Out.

> "Baby this town rips the bones from your back / It's a death trap, its a suicide rap / We gotta get out while we're young / cause tramps like us, baby we were born to run"
>
> Bruce Springsteen, Born To Run

Comments:

Annie A.

Ed, THANKS for picking my fav Bruce song! You are the epitome of grace and style during this whole journey! Very proud of you, and also Dad, Tom and Kathy for always being there for you! Reflect and relax knowing you won the battle and can plan on an awesome future! Love you Bro! xoxoxo

Uncle Bob

Hi Eddie, God is good and has answered your prayers and those of many. We are so happy for you as you have so much to offer in your caring and kind ways. Enjoy each day and continue to trust in His love! Uncle Bob and Aunt Kathy

Audrey J.

Take some time to think on it and then do whatever makes you happy :) You literally got a second chance!

Extended version:

The Cavaliers were still in the thick of the playoffs, and the whole city was buzzing with optimism over them. It seemed like a good time to close these journal entries on CaringBridge. The phrase, "Out," I borrowed from the slang used by Jim Rome and his audience, known as "The Jungle," which I enjoyed through my cable connection at home while I was out sick. He was no longer on terrestrial radio in Cleveland. 'Out' is used when Jim signs off of his show or when one of the more savvy clones (audience members) are through with their take (phone-in call).

This had been the longest four months of my life, and now it was over, so "Out" was as appropriate signature as any. The song from Bruce Springsteen had always been a Cleveland favorite. In its heyday during the seventies, local rocker, WMMS-FM, in Cleveland always played it at the end of the workday on Friday, signaling release! I thought it's be as good of a high energy tune as any to close out these journal entries.

And the Bible entry was totally appropriate and maybe convinced me that this should be the last entry. Like the phrase, "this week," which I still was using a lot; the phrase, "if the Lord is willing," would keep coming up when people would ask me if I would be continue teaching for Kent State on the side, if I planned to go back to biking, if I planned to travel to library conventions again, if…if…

Any question from friends, colleagues, and family about my old life before and new life after cancer, I had always framed in an optimistic tone. But when I saw this quote, it sealed the deal as far as my stock bullet point answer for any of these if-I-would questions. Saved my throat from exertion, saved time spent talking about something I couldn't really predict and was my own little prayer that I would share with them in hopes of being a good role model in faith. Something the good priests, nuns, and brothers in schools of my past would be proud of.

The quote from James 4:13–14 combines both the humbleness and optimism I felt as a cancer survivor. I would strive to recapture the best of the old life and look forward to these extra days I had. I was, indeed, a new man, older, wiser, and forty pounds lighter. But it had been the Lord who got me to this point, not my own discipline. And no matter what I'd plan to do next, I realized that it'd be the Lord's decision to let me proceed on this life's run. I might've been "born to run," but He holds the checkered flag!

Afterwards

I t would be about a month before I decided to retire. I gave two months' notice at the end of June. Fatigue was a major factor, driving forty minutes (on a good day) would tire me out like never before. Despite extra vitamins and doing protein shakes, I still had a lack of energy. The dry mouth I experienced caused me to wake up every couple of hours, unless I used a sleep aid, which I still treat myself to once a week, just to get five hours of straight sleep in.

I've used various remedies, omega-7, zinc, a humidifier in the room at night, and now a year later, still am glad when I can get four hours in without waking. Sometimes I get six in without doing anything unusual, so I guess it's like my dad said, "Healing is a slow process."

Management at Shaker had been great about giving me off the floor time, but I really didn't feel like I was pulling my own weight and wouldn't be for a while. Better to cut the cord and let them hire or promote someone else into the position who could go at it 100 percent.

Here was my retirement announcement for the staff at the library, paraphrasing lines from the end of the movie, *Pulp Fiction*.

VINCENT. So if you're retiring from the life at Shaker Library, what'll you do?

ED. That's what I've been sitting here contemplating. First, I'm gonna deliver this book to Marsellus. Then, basically, I'm gonna walk the earth.

VINCENT. What do you mean walk the earth?

ED. You know, like Caine in *Kung Fu*. Just walk from town to town, meet people, get in adventures.

VINCENT. How long do you intend to walk the earth?

ED. Until God puts me where He wants me to be.

VINCENT. What if he never does?

ED. If it takes forever, I'll wait forever.

I had the years in and was at the right age to draw a decent pension, and the windfall inheritance from Betty really made it possible. The month after retiring as executor I spent selling her house and settling the last of her estate details. I spent my birthday taking Kathy to see the Ark Encounter in Kentucky; something that had been on my bucket list, and that I'd encourage anyone to go see. I was hoping to do zip lining down on their property, which everyone told me NOT to do in my weakened, still healing condition. It ended up being a rainy day, so I wasn't tempted to try it.

This year...I'm staying involved with my industry but at my own pace. In October, hurricane Michael destroyed Panama City, where my sister lived. It prompted me to write an article called "Crisis Fund Raising in the era of Climate Change," combining various elements from my previously published book, *40+ New Revenue Sources for Libraries and Nonprofits*. I'm also giving presentations on my favorite author, Stephen King, at various local libraries and nursing homes. Played a few rounds of golf in the fall with my buddies and really felt blessed no matter how tough the round went. I was in the sun, free, and with my friends. Something was missing though.

Although I'd been responsible enough, I thought I should be doing more. I had a card from Sokolowski's University Inn, a great Polish restaurant in Cleveland going back to 1923. I received it from the owner at a party once years ago. There was a prayer on the back of it that related to retirement. It was so cool, I asked him for a stash of them and would give them to coworkers, friends, and patrons at the library when I heard of their retirement.

Prayer from Sokolowski's

Lord, keep me working, keep me fit
At windows I don't want to sit
Watching my fellows hurrying by
Let me stay busy till I die.
Grant me strength, breath and will
a need to serve and a task to do.
Let me each morning rise anew
Eager and glad that I can bear
My portion of the morning care.
Lord I don't want to sit about
Broken and tired and all worn out
Afraid of rain, and wind and cold,
Let me stay busy when I am old.
Although I walk at a slower pace
Still let me meet life face to face.
This is my prayer as time goes by
Lord keep me busy till I die.

One day, I noticed on my computer the bookmark for CaringBridge in my browser and went into it. Scrolling through the entries got me thinking about giving something back to all those who supported me. At first, I was thinking just a glorified version of it in a PDF for friends and family, but then thought perhaps I could do something more. Hopefully this manuscript sheds light on the throat cancer experience for both the patients and their caregivers. The original CaringBridge platform was called "The Rossman Rally," but since that's way too vague for a mass market, I figured "A Guy's Guide to Throat Cancer" would be a lot more descriptive. Ever the librarian, we are all about accessibility!

I hope it helps "rally" everyone reading to go the distance in your own personal struggles and to call on the Holy Trinity and all the angels and saints to give you strength and confidence to overcome cancer and live in gratitude through your actions.

Because, as the Grateful Dead sing about our lives in their song Box of Rain (our planet Earth) it's "such a long, long time to be gone and a short time to be there."

Keep the faith.

References

Backstory

AZ Quotes, "Kay Yow Quote-When life kicks you, let it kick you forward", accessed March 4, 2019, https://www.azquotes.com/quote/533972.

CaringBridge, "Ed Rossman—The Rossman Rally", January 20, 2018, accessed February 8, 2019, https://www.caringbridge.org/public/edrossman.

The Word Among Us Magazine can be found/contacted at www.wa.org, www.facebook.com/wordamongus, 1-800-775-WORD (9673) or via snail mail at

7115 Guilford Dr Ste 100
Frederick, MD 21704

Their motto, "A Daily Approach to Prayer and Scripture" was helpful in every way as I went through months at home not being able to go to church during my cancer treatment. Any mistakes on bible quotations in this book I totally blame on my Chemo brain!

Forward / January 20, 2018

Venuto, Tom. *Burn the fat, feed the muscle: transform your body forever using the secrets of the leanest people in the world.* New York. Harmony Books. 2013.

Journal 1—January 20, 2018

John Wooden Quotes. BrainyQuote.com, BrainyMedia Inc, 2019. https://www.brainyquote.com/quotes/john_wooden_446997, accessed May 1, 2019.

Wikipedia, "Pope Fabian", May 12, 2002, accessed March 4, 2019, https://en.wikipedia.org/wiki/Pope_Fabian.

Journal 2—January 22, 2018

National Cancer Institute, "Cisplatin", July 25, 2018, accessed February 28, 2019, https://www.cancer.gov/about-cancer/treatment/drugs/cisplatin

Thirty Seconds To Mars. "Walk On Water ". Filmed [July 2017]. You Tube video, 03:20. Posted [August 2017]. https://www.youtube.com/watch?v=FA2w-PMKspo

Journal 3—January 23, 2018

Journey. "Journey—Don't Stop Believin". [.] You Tube video, 04:10. Posted [April 2013]. https://www.youtube.com/watch?v=1k8craCGpgs

Radiological Society of North America, "IMRT-Intensity-Modulated Radiation Therapy", January 25, 2017, accessed February 28, 2019, https://www.radiologyinfo.org/en/info.cfm?pg=imrt.

Journal 4—January 25, 2018

Mandino, Og. *The Greatest Salesman in the World*. New York. Bantam Books. 1985.

Journal 5 January 28, 2018

Lou Holtz Quotes. BrainyQuote.com, BrainyMedia Inc, 2019.

https://www.brainyquote.com/quotes/lou_holtz_450770, accessed May 1, 2019

Tsakiris, Diomidis. "Mike Oldfield 'Tubular Bells' Live at the BBC 1973". Filmed [November 1973]. You Tube video, 25:46. Posted [January 2017]. https://www.youtube.com/watch?v=4nfaQb2r5QA.

Journal 7 February 2, 2018

Aquinas and more, "Peregrine Healing Relic Card", 2019, accessed March 1 2019, https://www.aquinasandmore.com/buy/peregrine-healing-relic-card-94560/.

Blues Traveler. "Blues Traveler—But Anyway". Filmed [1994]. You Tube video, 03:06. Posted [September 2010]. https://www.youtube.com/watch?v=XjYGpTkoRVw.

John Wooden Quotes. BrainyQuote.com, BrainyMedia Inc, 2019. https://www.brainyquote.com/quotes/john_wooden_446994, accessed May 1, 2019.

Parissa Janaraghi, "Saving Private Ryan Quotes", 2019, accessed March 1, 2019, https://www.moviequotesandmore.com/saving-private-ryan-quotes/.

Rossman, Edmund A, *40+ New Revenue Sources for Libraries and Nonprofits*, Chicago, ALA Editions, 2016.

Journal 8—February 4, 2018

Bonnat, Leon. *Job*. Accessed March 4, 2019. https://commons.wikimedia.org/w/index.php?curid=2188483

Lawrence OP. *St Blaise*. Accessed March 4, 2019. https://www.flickr.com/photos/paullew/32562213661

Coast Caritas. *St Peregrine*. Accessed March 4, 2019. https://coastcaritas.wordpress.com/2016/06/08/ novena-to-st-peregrine-for-my-uncles-pancreatic-cancer/

Wikipedia, "Peregrine Laziosi", January 23, 2006, accessed March 4, 2019, https://en.wikipedia.org/wiki/Peregrine_Laziosi.

Wikipedia, "Saint Blaise", February 4, 2004, accessed March 4, 2019, https://en.wikipedia.org/wiki/Saint_Blaise.

Journal 9—February 8, 2018

American Speech-Language-Hearing Association, "Adult Dysphagia Treatment", accessed March 6, 2019, https://www.asha.org/PRPSpecificTopic.aspx?folderid=8589942550 &section=Treatment

Bear Grylls Quotes. BrainyQuote.com, BrainyMedia Inc, 2019. https://www.brainyquote.com/quotes/bear_grylls_512952, accessed May 1, 2019.

CatholicSaints.Info, "Saint Jerome Emiliani",January 28, 2018, accessed March 6, 2019, http://catholicsaints.info/saint-jerome-emiliani/

Lyricsfreak, "Ac Dc Thunderstruck Lyrics", accessed March 23, 2019, https://www.lyricsfreak.com/a/ac+dc/thunderstruck_20003371.html

Mack, Carrie. "Military Montage to Thunderstruck". Filmed [.]. You Tube video, 04:51. Published [2015]. https://www.dailymotion.com/video/x2q631h.

Russell Simmons Quotes. BrainyQuote.com, BrainyMedia Inc, 2019. https://www.brainyquote.com/quotes/russell_simmons_219455, accessed May 1, 2019.

Journal 10—February 12, 2018

alwilbury. "Eric Clapton—Hello Old Friend (1976)". Filmed [.] You Tube video, 03:34. Posted [April 2011]. https://www.youtube.com/watch?v=XAZ5G3xoxhI

Stands4 LLC, "Hello Old Friend–Lyrics.com"., accessed March 23, 2019, https://www.lyrics.com/lyric/584722/Eric+Clapton/Hello+Old+Friend

Journal 11—February 14, 2018

Castaneda, Carlos. *The teachings of Don Juan: a Yaqui way of knowledge.* Berkeley. University of California Press. 1968.

Joel Osteen Quotes. BrainyQuote.com, BrainyMedia Inc, 2019. https://www.brainyquote.com/quotes/joel_osteen_579117, accessed May 1, 2019.

Ray, James. "San Jacinto by Peter Gabriel" Filmed [.]. You Tube video, 06:25. Posted [May 2016]. https://www.youtube.com/watch?v=ofxAXhlUXhM.

Songfacts, "San Jacinto by Peter Gabriel", 2019, accessed March 1 2019, https://www.songfacts.com/facts/peter-gabriel/san-jacinto

Wikipedia, "Ash Wednesday", January 17, 2003, accessed March 4, 2019, https://en.wikipedia.org/wiki/Ash_Wednesday.

Journal 12—February 18, 2018

AZ Quotes, "Kay Yow Quote-When life kicks you, let it kick you forward", accessed march 4, 2019, https://www.azquotes.com/quote/533972.

NickelCreekVEVO. "Nickel Creek—Smoothie Song." Filmed [.]. You Tube video, 03:42. Posted [May 2009]. https://www.youtube.com/watch?v=QcjAXI4jANw.

St. Francis Quote. Goodreades Endurance Quotes. Goodreads, Inc. 2019. https://www.goodreads.com/quotes/tag/endurance, accessed May 1, 2019.

Journal 13—February 25, 2018

tompetty. "Tom Petty And The Heartbreakers—The Waiting". Filmed [1981]. You Tube video, 04:19. Posted [October 2009]. https://www.youtube.com/watch?v=uMyCa35_mOg.

Wikipedia, "The Jim Rome Show", July 5, 2005, accessed March 5, 2019, https://en.wikipedia.org/wiki/The_Jim_Rome_Show

Journal 14—February 28, 2018

The Chemical Brothers. "The Chemical Brothers—Galvanize". Filmed [2005]. You Tube video, 03:43. Posted [July 2011]. https://www.youtube.com/watch?v=Xu3FTEmN-eg.

Derrick Brooks. AZQuotes.com, Wind and Fly LTD, 2019. https://www.azquotes.com/quote/1300884, accessed May 01, 2019.

Rodney Atkins. "If You're Going Through Hell (Official). Filmed[.]. You Tube Video, 03:42. Posted [September 2011]. https://www.youtube.com/watch?v=l50L4GYhpLc.

Wikipedia, "Krumping", October 12, 2018, accessed March 4, 2019, https://en.wikipedia.org/wiki/Krumping.

Journal 15—March 15, 2018

Brady, Tom. *The TB12 method: how to achieve a lifetime of sustained peak performance.* New York. Simon and Schuster. 2017.

Milford, Rob. "Pink Floyd—...home, home again...(Time)". Filmed [.]. You Tube video, 01:11. Posted [February 2014]. https://www.youtube.com/watch?v=KmKaomo5Y8Y.

Journal 16—March 16, 2018

Cahill, Thomas. *How the Irish saved civilization the untold story of Ireland's heroic role from the fall of Rome to the rise of medieval Europe.* Thorndike, Me. G.K. Hall. 1998.

KingxxCrusader. "Led Zeppelin—Lord of the Rings—Battle of Evermore—AMV". Filmed [.]. YouTube video, 05:49. Posted [November 2008]. https://www.youtube.com/watch?v=UUmd6lujmuE.

T.D. Jakes Quotes. oChristian.com, 2019. http://christian-quotes.ochristian.com/T.D.-Jakes-Quotes/page-4.shtml, accessed May 1, 2019

Wikimedia Commons. *Guido_Reni.jpg.* Image, 2012. https://en.wikipedia.org/wiki/File:Guido_Reni_031.jpg.

Wikipedia, "Prayer to Saint Michael", January 8, 2018, accessed March 4, 2019, https://en.wikipedia.org/wiki/Prayer_to_Saint_Michael.

Journal 17—March 14, 2018

Lord Byron Quotes. BrainyQuote.com, BrainyMedia Inc, 2019. https://www.brainyquote.com/quotes/lord_byron_378386, accessed May 1, 2019.

Timbuk3VEVO. "Timbuk 3—The Future's So Bright". Filmed [.]. You Tube video, 03:20. Posted [march 2009]. https://www.youtube.com/watch?v=8qrriKcwvlY.

Wikipedia, "The End (Beatles song)", March 28, 2005, accessed March 4, 2019, https://en.wikipedia.org/wiki/The_End_(Beatles_song).

Journal 18—March 19, 2018

Milo77ut. "R.E.M.—You Are the Everything". Filmed [.]. You Tube video, 03:44. Posted [March 2012]. https://www.youtube.com/watch?v=6e-LF21yFWM.

Pope Francis: 16 January 2015: Discourse to families in Manila. Dicasterium pro Communicatione.
https://www.vaticannews.va/en/pope/news/2018-03/pope-francis-st-joseph-5-anniversary-pontificate.html, accessed May 2, 2019.

St. Swithun's RC Church, "Daily Readings for March 19, 2018", March 19, 2018, accessed March 6, 2019, http://stswithuns.org.uk/event/dr-19032018.

The Work of God's Children. *St Joseph*. Accessed March 4, 2019. http://marysrosaries.com/collaboration/index.php?title=File:Saint_Joseph_010.jpg

Journal 19—April 4, 2018

The Prayer Shawl was sent to me by Cathy Hackney, a great friend of my sister Ann. Her St. Thomas Prayer Shawl Ministry was based out of St. Thomas by the Sea in Panama City Beach, FL, https://www.stthomasbytheseapcb.org/

The prayer was based on one written by Cathleen O'Meara Murtha, DW, which I found at http://shawlministry.com/prayers.htm

acidslovs. "Citizen King—Better Days". Filmed [.]. You Tube video, 03:37. Posted [October 2010]. https://www.youtube.com/watch?v=87nJoBSfQ_Q.

Journal 20—April 10, 2018

My colleague, Miss Virginia, a long-time children's librarian really made me laugh with her supply of jokes and silly Jell-O songs. I wasn't familiar with Shel Silverstein, but he looks like a great talent that'll be missed. The lyrics and his voice are all over the internet, and a good review of his life and "Squishy Touch" poem can be found here: https://www.writework.com/essay/shel-silverstein

Bruce Lee Quotes. BrainyQuote.com, BrainyMedia Inc, 2019. https://www.brainyquote.com/quotes/bruce_lee_153190, accessed May 2, 2019.

Catholic Digest, "St. Frances de Sales-We Shall Steer Safely", November 17, 2018, accessed March 4, 2019, http://www.catholicdigest.com/from-the-magazine/quiet-moment/st-francis-de-sales-we-shall-steer-safely/.

Sulock, Timmy Flyersguy. "Chicago—Feelin stronger everyday (lyrics in description) Filmed [.]. You Tube video, 04:12. Posted [August 2011]. https://www.youtube.com/watch?v=yhRjA_yZEHA.

Venuto, Tom. *Burn the fat, feed the muscle: transform your body forever using the secrets of the leanest people in the world.* New York. Harmony Books. 2013.

Journal 21—April 14, 2018

The Cockburn Project. "Bruce Cockburn-Songs-Lovers In A Dangerous Time"…accessed May 2, 2019, http://cockburnproject.net/songs&music/liadt.html

Mandino, Og. *The Greatest Salesman in the World.* New York. Bantam Books. 1985.

Stands4 LLC, "Peaches lyrics—Lyrics.com"., accessed March 23, 2019, https://www.lyrics.com/lyric/1646413/The+Presidents+of+the+United+States+of+America/Peaches

Telstratouchfone. "Peaches—The Presidents of the United States of America". Filmed [.]. You Tube video, 03:11. Posted [October 2006]. https://www.youtube.com/watch?v=wvAnQqVJ3XQ.

Journal 22—April 22, 2018

60s70sVintageRock. "Chambers Brothers—Time Has Come Today (Live extended version)". Filmed [1969]. You Tube video, 14:54. Posted [December 2011]. https://www.youtube.com/watch?v=CsBwBct0_5U.

Reddit, Inc. "Do what you should do" https://www.reddit.com/r/inspiration/comments/a5avay/do_what_you_should_do_when_you_should_do_it/, accessed May 2, 2019.

Stands4 LLC, "Time Has Come Today lyrics—Lyrics.com," accessed March 23, 2019, https://www.lyrics.com/lyric/125359/The+Chambers+Brothers/Time+Has+Come+Today

Journal 23—April 26, 2018

Castaneda, Carlos. *The fire from within.* New York. Simon and Schuster. 1984.

Kosar, Bernie. *Learning to Scramble.* University Heights, OH. Cleveland Landmarks Press, Inc. 2017. p. 12
Nine Inch Nails. "Nine Inch Nails—We're In This Together". Filmed [1999]. You Tube video, 06:18. Posted [June 2009]. https://www.youtube.com/watch?v=P9BfvPjsXXw.

Journal 24—May 1, 2018

Grateful Dead. "Grateful Dead—Touch Of Grey (Official Music Video)". Filmed [1987]. You Tube video, 04:52. Posted [September 2012]. https://www.youtube.com/watch?v=mzvk0fWtCs0.

Stands4 LLC, "Touch of Grey lyrics—Lyrics.com"., accessed March 23, 2019, https://www.lyrics.com/lyric/2007084/grateful+dead/touch+of+grey

Journal 25—May 6, 2018

Colonel Parker. "Carry On My Wayward Son Kansas Lyrics". Filmed [.]. You Tube video, 05:28. Posted [November 2013]. https://www.youtube.com/watch?v=pkjKAZ70jzk.

Mayo Clinic, "CT Scan", accessed March 5, 2019, https://www.mayoclinic.org/tests-procedures/ct-scan/about/pac-20393675

Journal 26—May 13, 2018

Chadman2000. "Rare Earth—I Just Want To Celebrate". Filmed [.]. You Tube video, 03:45. Posted [March 2008]. https://www.youtube.com/watch?v=VRVPLPFoJL0.

PJ McIntyres' Irish Pub, accessed March 22, 2019, http://pjmcintyres.com/

WebMD, "Laryngoscopy-Purpose, Procedures, Types and Comp lications", accessed March 5, 2019, https://www.webmd.com/oral-health/what-is-laryngoscopy#2

Journal 27—May 23, 2018

Anner92. "Bruce Springsteen—Born To Run". Filmed [.]. You Tube video, 04:31. Posted [November 2008]. https://www.youtube.com/watch?v=f3t9SfrfDZM.

Wikipedia, "The Jim Rome Show", July 5, 2005, accessed March 5, 2019, https://en.wikipedia.org/wiki/The_Jim_Rome_Show

Afterwards—Summer, 2018

American Library Association, "40+ New Revenue Sources for Libraries and Nonprofits, 2016, accessed March 5, 2019, https://www.alastore. ala.org/content/40-new-revenue-sources-libraries-and-nonprofits

Answers In Genesis, "Ark Encounter", 2019, accessed March 5, 2019, https://arkencounter.com/

Blacktext. "Pulp Fiction (1994)—The coffee shop conversation", August 2007, accessed March 5, 2019, https://blacktext.wordpress. com/2007/08/04/pulp-fiction-1994-the-coffee-shop-conversation/

Box Of Rain was written by Philip Lesh and Robert C. Hunter of the Grateful Dead, legend has it as Phil Lesh's father was dying and he was taking care of him. The last line is a fitting coda to a book about living through cancer, IMHO. https://en.wikipedia.org/wiki/Box_of_Rain

LinkedIn, "Crisis Fundraising in the era of Climate Change", November 20, 2018,accessed March 5, 2019, https://www.linkedin. com/pulse/crisis-fundraising-era-climate-change-ed-rossman/

Robert Kennedy.

http://3.bp.blogspot.com/_z535W0Oeans/SfnxNtH1hmI/AAAAAAAA AEg/0nbWhesx83I/s400/pulp10807sk.jpg,Image,.http://cranesareflying1. blogspot.com/2012/12/pulp-fiction.html

Sokolowski's, "Sokolowski's University Inn", 2015, accessed March 5, 2019, https://www.sokolowskis.com/

Index of Bible References

OLD TESTAMENT

Journal 1

"The Lord granted him a stern struggle, that he might know that godliness is more powerful than anything else." Wisdom 10:12

Journal 8

"I, too, have been assigned months of futility, long, and weary nights of misery." Job 7:3

Journal 15

"Yea, though I walk through the valley of the shadow of death, I will fear no evil: for thou art with me; thy rod and thy staff they comfort me..." Psalm 23:4

Journal 20

"For everything there is a season, and a time for every matter under heaven" Ecclesiastes 3:1

Journal 22

"How shall I make a return to the Lord for all the good he has done for me?" Psalm 116:12

Journal 24

"Let your eyes look straight ahead, and your gaze be focused forward." Proverbs 4:25

Journal 25

"The steps of a good man are ordered by the LORD: and He delighteth in his way. Though he fall, he shall not be utterly cast down: for the LORD upholdeth him with his hand." Psalm 37:23–24

NEW TESTAMENT

Journal 2

"Why did you lose faith?" Matthew 14:22–34

Journal 5

"For God did not give us a spirit of cowardice but rather of power and love and self-control." 2 Timothy 1:7

Journal 10

"Consider it all joy, my brothers and sisters, when you encounter various trials, for you know that the testing of your faith produces perseverance" James 1:2–3

Journal 15

"but whoever drinks of the water that I will give him shall never thirst; but the water that I will give him will become in him a well of water springing up to eternal life." John 4:14

Journal 23

"But the fruit of the Spirit is love, joy, peace, forbearance, kindness, goodness, faithfulness, gentleness, and self-control. Against such things, there is no law." Galatians 5:22–23

Journal 23

"Do not regard lightly the discipline of the Lord, nor lose courage when you are punished by him. For the Lord disciplines him who he loves" Hebrews 12:5–6

Journal 26

"May the God of hope fill you with all joy and peace in believing, so that by the power of the Holy Spirit you may abound in hope." Romans 15:13

Journal 27

Come now, you who say, "Today or tomorrow we will go to this or that city, spend a year there, carry on business, and make a profit." You do not even know what will happen tomorrow! What is your life? You are a mist that appears for a little while and then vanishes. Instead, you ought to say, "If the Lord is willing, we will live and do this or that." James 4:13–14

Mixtape for A Guy's Guide to Throat Cancer

Tunes used in quotes or videos in my CaringBridge entries:

Gimme Shelter (extended version) by The Rolling Stones—Backstory
Walk on Water by Thirty Seconds to Mars—Journal 2
Don't Stop Believin' by Journey—Journal 3
Supper's Ready by Genesis—Journal 3
Lincoln Portrait by Aaron Copland—Journal 3
Tubular Bells by Mike Oldfield—Journal 5
But Anyway by Blues Traveler—Journal 7
Various greatest hits by Yes and Genesis—Journal 7
Thunderstruck by AC/DC—Journal 9
Hello Old Friend by Eric Clapton—Journal 10
San Jacinto by Peter Gabriel—Journal 11
Smoothie Song by Nickel Creek—Journal 12
The Waiting by Tom Petty and the Heartbreakers—Journal 13
Galvanize by The Chemical Brothers—Journal 14
If You're Going Through Hell by Rodney Atkins—Journal 14
Time by Pink Floyd—Journal 15
No Quarter by Led Zeppelin Journal 15
Battle of Evermore by Led Zeppelin—Journal 16
The Future's So Bright by Timbuk 3—Journal 17
The End by The Beatles—Journal 17
You Are the Everything by R.E.M.—Journal 18
Better Days by Citizen King—Journal 19

Feelin' Stronger Everyday by Chicago—Journal 20
Squishy Touch by Shel Silverstein—Journal 20
Lovers In A Dangerous Time by Bruce Cockburn—Journal 21
Peaches by Presidents Of The United States—Journal 21
Time Has Come Today by The Chambers Brothers—Journal 22
We're In This Together by Nine Inch Nails—Journal 23
Touch of Grey by The Grateful Dead—Journal 24
Carry On My Wayward Son by Kansas—Journal 25
I Just Want To Celebrate by Rare Earth—Journal 26
Born To Run by Bruce Springsteen—Journal 27
Box of Rain by The Grateful Dead—Afterwards

About the Author

E dmund A. Rossman III has been involved with libraries and broadcasting since 1980. After surviving cancer he retired from the Shaker Heights Public Library (OH) in 2018. He is the author of Castles Against Ignorance: How to Make Libraries Great Educational Environments (2006) and 40+ New Revenue Sources for Libraries and Nonprofits (2016). He has taught courses for Kent State University in Journalism and Library Science. Currently he does eCourses and webinars nationally on fundraising. He also does local presentations on his favorite author, Stephen King, in libraries and nursing homes using his own photography of book settings. As a business manager of radio stations in two major markets, he coordinated dozens of sponsorship campaigns, as well as produced over 200 hours of award-winning specialty programming. He graduated from Cleveland State University with a BA in Communications. He holds Masters degrees in Communications from Ohio University and in Library and Information Science from Kent State University.

CPSIA information can be obtained
at www.ICGtesting.com
Printed in the USA
LVHW051347210520
656048LV00002B/251